Women's Neurology

What Do I Do Now?

SERIES CO-EDITORS-IN-CHIEF

Lawrence C. Newman, MD
Director of the Headache Institute
Department of Neurology
St. Luke's-Roosevelt Hospital Center
New York, New York

Morris Levin, MD
Codirector of the Dartmouth Headache Center
Director of the Dartmouth Neurology Residency Training Program
Section of Neurology
Dartmouth Hitchcock Medical Center
Lebanon, New Hampshire

OTHER VOLUMES IN THE SERIES

Women's Neurology

Edited by
M. Angela O'Neal
Department of Neurology
Harvard Medical School
Brigham and Women's Hospital
Boston, Massachusetts

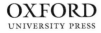

OXFORD
UNIVERSITY PRESS

OXFORD
UNIVERSITY PRESS

Oxford University Press is a department of the University of Oxford. It furthers
the University's objective of excellence in research, scholarship, and education
by publishing worldwide. Oxford is a registered trade mark of Oxford University
Press in the UK and certain other countries.

Published in the United States of America by Oxford University Press
198 Madison Avenue, New York, NY 10016, United States of America.

CIP data is on file at the Library of Congress
ISBN 978–0–19–060991–7

9 8 7 6 5 4 3 2 1

Printed by WebCom, Inc., Canada

Contents

Preface

I wanted to write a book that addressed the common problems clinicians face in caring for women with neurological disorders. The gender-specific neurological issues clearly vary at different points in a woman's life. For example, these issues might include questions about reproductive health, pregnancy, or healthy aging. The book's raison d'être is to heighten caregivers' awareness about the gender differences in neurological care. A range of topics about women's health and neurological disorders is discussed, including: headache, stroke, epilepsy, neuropathy, Parkinson's disease, and Alzheimer's disease. The case scenarios are illustrative of common dilemmas we all face in caring for female patients. The discussions weigh the evidence available to help us make informed decisions with the best information on the particular topic. The cases are meant to demonstrate a best-practice clinical algorithm.

Topics covered in the book include issues that are unique to women, as well as those that may affect both men and women, but may have a different risk, prevalence, presentation, or treatment considerations for women. The book's format is based on the "What Do I Do Now?" texts, using case examples of common problems and questions that involve women with neurological disease and discussing how to best address the key issues. The aim is to give practical advice for everyday problems clinicians face in caring for women.

There is a lack of knowledge about how sex and gender may affect neurological illnesses. In addition, much of the research in this area is emerging or not widely publicized. Therefore, it can be challenging for physicians to stay on top of the latest research about how sex and gender affect the course of specific diseases, medication effects, and best neurological care. The book is meant to be a "go-to" manual to delineate best practices in women's neurology. It is written in a succinct straightforward style with tables, figures, and references illustrating the key clinical points. This book is unique as it addresses neurological problems women face throughout their lives, whereas previous texts in this area have been limited to neurological disorders that occur in pregnancy. The case-oriented format addressing the common clinical scenarios makes the book practical, relevant, and easy to read.

I hope you will enjoy reading the cases and working through the decision analyses. The authors did a great job in clarifying the dilemmas we all face on a regular basis in patient care. I know your female patients will benefit from the additional knowledge and expertise you gain after reading *Women's Neurology*.

—*Angela O'Neal, MD*

Contributors

Regina Krel, MD
Angels Neurological Centers, PC
Brighton, Massachusetts

Paul G. Mathew, MD, FAAN, FAHS
John R. Graham Headache Center
Department of Neurology
Brigham and Women's Hospital
Harvard Vanguard Medical Associates
Cambridge Health Alliance
Harvard Medical School
Boston, Massachusetts

Tamara B. Kaplan, MD
Partners Multiple Sclerosis Center
Department of Neurology
Brigham and Women's Hospital
Boston, Massachusetts

Marcelo Matiello, MD, MSc
Department of Neurology
Massachusetts General Hospital
Harvard Medical School
Boston, Massachusetts

Chizoba Umeh, MD
Department of Neurology
Brigham and Women's Hospital
Boston, Massachusetts

Eudocia Q. Lee, MD, MPH
Center for Neuro-Oncology
Dana Farber Cancer Institute
Brigham and Women's Hospital
Boston, Massachusetts

Alexandra Lovett, MD
Department of Neurology
Massachusetts General Hospital
Brigham and Women's Hospital
Boston, Massachusetts

Whitney Woodmansee, MD
Department of Endocrinology
Brigham and Women's Hospital
Boston, Massachusetts

P. Emanuela Voinescu, MD, PhD
Department of Neurology
Epilepsy Division
Brigham and Women's Hospital
Boston, Massachusetts

Janet Waters, MD, MBA
Women's Neurology
Magee Women's Hospital
University of Pittsburgh
Medical Center
Pittsburgh, Pennsylvania

Marie Pasinski, MD
Department of Neurology
Harvard Medical School
Charlestown HealthCare Center
Massachusetts General Hospital
Charlestown, Massachusetts

Sandra L. Horowitz, MD
Department of Neurology
Brigham and Women's Hospital
Boston, Massachusetts

Na Tosha N. Gatson, MD, PhD
Department of Neurology
Geisinger Health System
Danville, Pennsylvania

Terri L. Woodard, MD
Department of Gynecologic
   Oncology
Reproductive Medicine
University of Texas
MD Anderson Cancer Center
Houston, Texas

Issues in Women During Their Reproductive Years

1 Hormonal Contraception in a Woman with Headache

M. Angela O'Neal

A 27-year-old woman comes for evaluation of long-standing headaches. She reports the headaches began in high school, and are usually right hemicranial and throbbing in nature. They are often preceded by shimmering zigzag lines, which occur out of the right side of her vision. These visual phenomena are often followed by a right visual field loss. The visual symptoms typically last about 20–30 minutes. The headaches are associated with light sensitivity as well as nausea and vomiting. They occur at least once a week and last 24–48 hours. She has previously tried amitriptyline, propranolol, and Excedrin migraine tablets without success. She has not noticed any clear triggers for her headaches.

Her past medical history is unremarkable.

Her current medications are Ortho-Tri-Cyclen and naproxen PRN (i.e., as needed). She drinks alcohol occasionally and smokes cigarettes, about one pack a day.

Her examination is normal.

What do you do now?

MIGRAINE AND HORMONAL CONTRACEPTION

Diagnosis

This lady suffers from migraine with aura. The diagnosis of migraine with aura can be confidently made on a clinical history based on the International Headache Society (IHS) criteria for migraine with aura shown in Box 1.1. Patients with a new presentation of probable migraine with aura need imaging, usually a brain magnetic resonance image (MRI) and neck and brain vascular imaging to exclude secondary headaches that can mimic migraine.

Migraine has been reported to affect as many as 43% of women in the United States. The prevalence of migraine increases with age such that in the 35–39-year age bracket, as many as 37% of women may be affected. The prevalence of migraine with aura is 4.4%.[1] Combined hormonal contraception (CHC) is the most commonly prescribed method of contraception. A US Health and Human Services survey from 2006–2008 found that 10.4 million women ages 15–44 used an oral contraceptive pill (OCP).[2] Therefore, choosing the appropriate candidate for this method is important. There are several significant issues in choosing an appropriate contraceptive method in women who have migraine with aura. These concerns include: the risk of stroke with CHCs, the risk of stroke in migraineurs with aura, and choosing the appropriate contraception method for a

---

BOX 1.1 **IHS Diagnostic Criteria for Migraine with Aura**

Must fulfill criteria for migraine listed above, and in addition, at least two attacks fulfilling the following criteria.
  Aura consisting of at least one of the following, but no motor weakness:

1. Fully reversible visual symptoms, including positive features (flickering lights, spots, or lines) and/or negative features (i.e., loss of vision)
2. Fully reversible sensory symptoms, including positive features and/or negative features
3. Fully reversible dysphasic speech disturbance

At least two of the following other characteristics:

1. Homonymous visual symptoms and/or unilateral sensory symptoms
2. At least one aura symptom develops gradually over ≥ 5 min, and/or different aura symptoms occur in succession over ≥ 5 min
3. Each symptom lasts ≥ 5 and < 60 min

Headache fulfilling the criteria for migraine without aura begins during the aura or follows aura within 60 minutes the headache disorder.

---

patient for whom we want to start prophylactic migraine treatment, which may have a teratogenic risk.

Stroke Risk and Oral Contraceptive Pills

The absolute risk for ischemic stroke (IS) in women using a CHC is small, but it rises dramatically after age 45. The risk is exclusively related to estrogen, and there has been no evidence to suggest progesterone alone confers additional risk. A meta-analysis of studies showed 2.75 greater odds of a stroke in a woman with any OCP use.[3] More recent studies looking exclusively at low-dose CHCs have shown a comparable risk. The data for hemorrhagic stroke risk are less consistent. It is known that the risk of stroke with OCPs increases in women who have other traditional stroke risk factors, such as increased age, smoking, hypertension or taking estrogen-containing contraceptives. For these women, CHCs may not be the best choice of contraception, and aggressive stroke risk-factor modification is important.[4]

Stroke Risk in Migraine with Aura

The absolute risk of IS is small. The Women's Health Study (WHS) found that there were four additional cases of IS per 10,000 women each year where migraine with aura was the presumed etiology. This study also showed that migraineurs with aura tended to have transient ischemic attacks and non-disabling strokes. An increased frequency of migraine with aura is associated with an increased risk of stroke.[5] Therefore, the American Heart Association in its guidelines on stroke in women recommends that prophylactic medication should be considered in women who have frequent migraine with aura. In addition, smoking cessation is strongly recommended.[6]

Oral Contraceptive Pills' Interactions with Migraine Medications

Practically speaking, medication interaction with OCPs is not significant for most medications used for acute or abortive therapy unless these medications are being used in excess. When prescribing a medication for a woman in the childbearing years, the medication safety during pregnancy should be considered. If the medication to be prescribed has potentially teratogenic effects, then other effective contraception should be discussed. In addition, what effect, if any, the medication may have on their current mode of contraception should also be considered. Table 1.1 shows the common classes of medication used for migraine prophylaxis and their pregnancy classification. Table 1.2 shows the effects of common migraine prophylactic medications on OCPs. For the most part, there are no significant interactions except when topiramate is used in doses above 200 mg daily.

TABLE 1.1 Migraine Preventative Medications and Level of Risk During Pregnancy

Drug Class	Generic Name	Level of Risk During Pregnancy
Beta blockers	Atenolol	D
	Nadolol, Propranolol, Metoprolol	C (D at term)
Antiepileptics	Gabapentin	C
	Topirimate	C
	Valproate	D
Calcium channel blocker	Verapamil	C
Tricyclic antidepressants	Amitriptyline	C

Recommendations to our patient would be:

1. She should discontinue the CHC and use either a non-hormonal or a progesterone-only contraceptive method. One highly effective and appropriate contraceptive for this type of patient is the Mirena intrauterine device (IUD).
2. Given her small but real risk from stroke due to migraine with aura, smoking cessation should be strongly recommended.
3. Prophylactic medication should be offered to her due to the frequency of her migraines. Topiramate would be a reasonable choice. The doses used in migraine prophylaxis would not interfere with her contraception

TABLE 1.2 Commonly Used Migraine Preventative Medications and OCP Interaction

Drug Class	Generic name	OCP Interaction
Beta blockers	Atenolol, Propranolol	No effect
Antiepileptics	Gabapentin	No effect
	Topiramate	Decreases efficacy in doses > 200 mg/d
	Valproate	No effect
Calcium channel blocker	Verapamil	No effect
Tricyclic antidepressants	Amitriptyline	No effect

method. However, a discussion about why an effective contraceptive method is needed is important, as topiramate is a pregnancy class D medication.

4. Abortive therapy with a triptan would also be appropriate.
5. She should initiate a headache diary to follow her migraine frequency and identify triggers, which would be discussed at her follow-up evaluation.

KEY POINTS TO REMEMBER

1. There is a small risk of stroke related to OCPs that is attributed to estrogen.
2. The risk of stroke related to CHCs increases with age and other traditional stroke risk factors; so, for women over the age of 45, especially with other stroke risk factors, another form of contraception should be considered.
3. Migraine with aura increases the risk of IS by 2.5 times, but the absolute number of strokes is small.
4. For women who have migraine with aura, CHCs should be avoided.

References

1. Stewart WF, Wood C, Reed ML, et al. Cumulative lifetime migraine incidence in women and men. *Cephalalgia*. 2008;28:1170–1178.
2. Mosher, WD. Use of contraception in the United States: 1982–2008. *Vital Health Stat*. 2010;23(29):1–44.
3. Gillum LA, BA, Mamidipudi SK, Johnston SC. Ischemic stroke risk with oral contraceptives: a meta-analysis. *JAMA*. 2000;284(1):72–78.
4. Lidegaard O, Løkkegaard E, Jensen A, et al. Thrombotic stroke and myocardial infarction with hormonal contraception. *NEJM*. 2012;366:2257–2266.
5. Spector JT, Kahn SR, Jones MR, et al. Migraine headache and ischemic stroke risk: an updated meta-analysis. *Am J Med*. 2010;123(7):612–624.
6. Bushnell C, McCullough LD, Awad IA, et al. Guidelines for the prevention of stroke in women. *Stroke*. 2014;45(5):1545–1588.

2 A Young Woman with Jerking Movements

M. Angela O'Neal

A 20-year-old lady presents for evaluation of seizures. She has had episodic jerking movements over the past year, which have increased over the last several months. She has fallen twice when the jerks involved her legs. They seem to be correlated with times when she gets poor sleep. She was recently seen in the emergency department (ED) after blacking out. She had stayed up late studying for a final. She woke to go to the bathroom, experienced several of these jerks, and then blacked out. Her roommate found her on the floor and called an ambulance. She denied any tongue bite or incontinence, but did admit to being generally sore and "foggy" when she woke up. The ED physician ordered a brain MRI, which was normal, and an electroencephalogram (EEG).

She has anxiety and depression.

Medications: fluoxetine 20 mg daily and a combined hormonal contraceptive.

On exam, height is 66 inches and weight is 200 lbs. Her neurological exam is normal. A sample portion of her EEG is shown in Figure 2.1.

What do you do now?

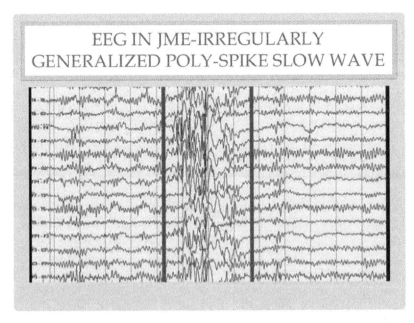

FIGURE 2.1 AP Bipolar montage showing typical high-voltage generalized 3–4 Hz spike polyspike wave characteristic for JME.

ANTICONVULSANTS AND HORMONAL CONTRACEPTION

This woman has juvenile myoclonic epilepsy (JME). This is one of the most common forms of generalized epilepsy, accounting for up to 25–30% of all idiopathic generalized epilepsy.[1] It is characterized by the triad of myoclonic jerks, generalized tonic clonic epilepsy, and absence seizures. Seizures typically occur in the morning and, as with this patient, are often triggered by sleep deprivation. In JME, the myoclonic jerks are epileptic. In general, JME is usually well controlled with medication, but most patients require lifelong anticonvulsant therapy.

Treatment for JME is with antiepileptic drugs (AEDs), which are effective for primary generalized epilepsy. In choosing an AED for a young woman of reproductive age, there are multiple considerations besides the efficacy of the medication. Some of these considerations include: the effect of an AED on her other medical conditions, potential medication interactions, long-term side effects, and teratogenic risk during pregnancy. In the context of our patient, there are several potentially efficacious medications. Let's weigh the choices.

Valproate is the best-studied and recommended first-line medication to treat JME. In one study for idiopathic generalized epilepsy, remission was seen in 52% of patients treated with valproate monotherapy, 17% for lamotrigine, and 34.6% for topiramate. Other studies have demonstrated that levetiracetam may be as effective as valproate in treating JME. Zonisemide may also be an effective AED in treating generalized epilepsy, but this is less well documented.[2]

Box 2.1 shows the potential interactions with each AED used for primary generalized epilepsy and combined hormonal contraceptives (CHCs).

Side effects to be considered for our patient include weight gain and exacerbation of her mood disorder. Valproate would not worsen her mood disorder, but weight gain, hair loss, and polycystic ovarian syndrome are known side effects. Lamotrigine, levetiracetam, and zonisamide are weight-neutral, whereas topiramate often causes weight loss. Levetiracetam can worsen anxiety, and topiramate in doses used to treat epilepsy may cause cognitive slowing.

There are considerable data documenting the teratogenic side effects of valproate, as well as long-term effects on fetal cognitive development. Therefore, despite its efficacy, it may not be the first choice of medication for women of reproductive age with JME. Topiramate is also a known teratogen. After a discussion with the patient, it was agreed to initiate levetiracetam.[3]

Table 2.1 shows each AEDs' pregnancy classification.

Levetiracetam was initiated, which controlled her JME. However, her anxiety worsened, so lamotrigine was gradually up-titrated and levetiracetam withdrawn.

Folate supplementation was begun at the time of the AED initiation. WWE have about twice the risk of neural tube defects, NTDs. Maternal folate deficiency has been linked with the development of NTDs, and periconceptional folate supplementation with a reduction of risk. It is not clear whether folate supplementation has a comparable protective effect for WWE. The American Academy of Neurology recommends the administration of 1–4 mg of folate for all WWE of child bearing potential.[4]

TABLE 2.1 **AEDs Used for Primary Generalized
Epilepsy Pregnancy Classification**

AED	Pregnancy Classification
Valproate	D
Topiramate	D
Lamotrigine	C
Levetiracetam	C
Zonisamide	C (fewer data available)

She was educated about the role of sleep deprivation as an epilepsy trigger, instructed as to safety concerns, and told not to drive for six months.

KEY POINTS TO REMEMBER

1. Valproate is the most effective AED for JME.
2. Due to concerns about valproate teratogenicity in a woman of reproductive age, other options should be considered.
3. The effect of an AED on metabolism of CHC needs to be considered and discussed.
4. Women with epilepsy in the childbearing years on an AED should also be taking folate supplementation.

References

1. Hauser WA. The prevalence and incidence of convulsive disorders in children. *Epilepsia*. 1994;35(Suppl 2):S1–S6.
2. Nicolson A, Appleton RE, Chadwick DW, Smith DF. The relationship between treatment with valproate, lamotrigine, and topiramate and the prognosis of the idiopathic generalized epilepsies. *J Neurol Neurosurg Psychiatry*. 2004; Jan;75(1):75–79.
3. Harden CL, Meador KJ, Pennell P, et al. Practice parameter update: management issues for women with epilepsy—focus on pregnancy (an evidence-based review): teratogenesis and perinatal outcomes: report of the Quality Standards Subcommittee and Therapeutics and Technology Assessment Subcommittee of the American Academy of Neurology and American Epilepsy Society. *Neurology*. 2009 Jul 14;73(2):133–141.
4. Morrell MJ. Folic Acid and Epilepsy. *Epilepsy Curr*. 2002 Mar;2(2):31–34.

3 Headache

Regina Krel and Paul G. Mathew

A 26-year-old female presents with throbbing unilateral headaches with an 8/10 intensity. They are associated with photophobia, phonophobia, nausea, and vomiting. She denies visual, sensory, language, or motor disturbances suggesting aura.

Individual attacks last 6–24 hours, and she estimates having seven headache days per month that tend to have a strong menstrual association. The majority of headaches begin two days prior to the onset of her menstrual cycle, and continue three days into menstruation. Her menstrual cycles are regular, occurring at 28-day intervals.

She has no other medical problems, and is not taking any medications. She has no allergies, and denies any tobacco or illicit drug use. There is a family history of migraines involving her mother and maternal grandmother. Her neurological examination was unremarkable.

What do you do now?

MENSTRUALLY RELATED MIGRAINE

At first glance, her diagnosis is seemingly obvious: migraine. The description of her headache fulfills criteria for episodic migraine without aura.[1] Migraines that have a menstrual association are further classified as pure menstrual migraine without aura, or menstrually related migraine without aura (Box 3.1). In this case, the patient has menstrually related migraine without aura, as this patient experiences some migraines outside of her menstrual periods.

The prevalence of menstrually related migraine can range from 20–60%, while pure menstrual migraine occurs in less than 10% of women.[8] Menstrual migraine attacks are typically not associated with aura symptoms. They tend to be more severe, longer lasting, more resistant to treatment, and associated with higher rates of functional disability.[2]

A diary documenting migraines and menstrual cycles should be kept over the course of three consecutive cycles. A diagnosis of menstrually related migraine can be confirmed when two of those menstrual cycles correlate with migraine onset within –2 to +3 days of menses. In contrast to sufferers of pure menstrual migraine, menstrually related migraine patients also have attacks at other points in their cycle.

Studies evaluating the relationship between the onset of migraine attack and its correlation to menstruation demonstrated a strong association with the natural

---

BOX 3.1 Diagnostic Criteria for Menstrual Migraine

PURE MENSTRUAL MIGRAINE WITHOUT AURA

Diagnostic criteria:

A. Attacks, in a menstruating woman, fulfilling criteria for Migraine without aura and criterion B below
B. Documented and prospectively recorded evidence over at least three consecutive cycles has confirmed that attacks occur exclusively on day 1 +/– 2 (i.e., days –2 to +3) of menstruation in at least two out of three menstrual cycles and at no other times of the cycle.

MENSTRUALLY RELATED MIGRAINE WITHOUT AURA

Diagnostic criteria:

A. Attacks, in a menstruating woman, fulfilling criteria for Migraine without aura and criterion B below
B. Documented and prospectively recorded evidence over at least three consecutive cycles has confirmed that attacks occur on day 1+/– 2 (i.e., days –2 to +3) of menstruation in at least two out of three menstrual cycles, and additionally at other times of the cycle.

---

drop in estrogen during the late luteal phase of the menstrual cycle. For women who have regular cycles and in whom a diagnosis of menstrually related migraine has been made, spot prophylactic or perimenstrual prophylactic treatment may be indicated. Prophylactic options can include nonsteroidal anti-inflammatory drugs (NSAIDs), triptans, and hormonal options.[5,6,7]

Medication dosage options include:[8]

- Naproxen sodium 550 mg twice daily for 5–14 days, starting the week before anticipated period onset.
- Frovatriptan to be started two days before period onset, with 5 mg taken twice daily on day 1, then 2.5 mg twice daily for six days.
- Naratriptan 1 mg twice daily for six days to be started three days before period onset.
- Zolmitriptan 2.5 mg twice or three times daily for seven days starting two days before expected period onset.

Hormonal options, such as estrogen supplementation, are geared to maintaining steady levels of estrogen, thus forestalling the abrupt drop that occurs during the late luteal phase. Since estrogen-based contraceptives are associated with an increased risk of stroke, and patients who suffer from migraine with aura carry a slightly increased risk of stroke, physicians should consider the use of progesterone-only formulations.

KEY POINTS TO REMEMBER

- Menstrually related migraines tend to be longer lasting, more debilitating, and more resistant to standard acute treatments than non-menstrual migraines.
- The diagnosis of menstrual migraine is made based on history, physical examination, and analysis of headache diaries demonstrating a menstrual relationship to headache in two out of three menstrual cycles. This diagnosis should be made after secondary headaches have been ruled out.
- Pathophysiology of menstrual migraine is thought to be related to the abrupt drop in estrogen in the late luteal phase and an increase in prostaglandins.
- Perimenstrual prophylaxis with NSAIDs, triptans, or hormones may be beneficial in reducing frequency and intensity of menstrually related migraine attacks.

References

1. Headache Classification Committee of the International Headache Society (IHS). *The International Classification of Headache Disorders*, 3rd edition (beta version). *Cephalalgia*. 2013;33(9):629–808. doi:10.1177/0333102413485658

2. Mathew PG, Dun EC, Luo JJ. A cyclic pain. *Obstet Gynecol Surv*. 2013;68(2):130–140. doi:10.1097/ogx.0b013e31827f2496

3. MacGregor EA, Victor TW, Hu X, et al. Characteristics of menstrual vs nonmenstrual migraine: a post hoc, within-woman analysis of the usual-care phase of a nonrandomized menstrual migraine clinical trial. *Headache*. 2010;50(4):528–538. doi:10.1111/j.1526-4610.2010.01625.x

4. Vetvik KG, Benth JS, Macgregor EA, Lundqvist C, Russell MB. Menstrual versus non-menstrual attacks of migraine without aura in women with and without menstrual migraine. *Cephalalgia*. 2015;35(14):1261–1268. doi:10.1177/0333102415575723

5. Macgregor EA, Frith A, Ellis J, Aspinall L, Hackshaw A. Prevention of menstrual attacks of migraine: a double-blind placebo-controlled crossover study. *Neurology*. 2006;67(12):2159–2163. doi:10.1212/01.wnl.0000249114.52802.55

6. Brandes J, Poole A, Kallela M, et al. Short-term frovatriptan for the prevention of difficult-to-treat menstrual migraine attacks. *Cephalalgia*. 2009;29(11):1133–1148. doi:10.1111/j.1468-2982.2009.01840.x

7. Macgregor EA. Contraception and headache. *Headache*. 2013;53(2):247–276. doi:10.1111/head.12035

8. Macgregor EA. Migraine management during menstruation and menopause. *Continuum*. 2015;21:990–1003. doi:10.1212/con.0000000000000196

4   Seeing Spots

Regina Krel and Paul G. Mathew

A 37-year-old female presents to the emergency department complaining of right arm numbness and tingling as well as seeing flashing spots and lines, which have persisted for two hours. She was in her usual state of health until two hours ago, when she noticed these symptoms. She has a history of migraine with visual aura, but her visual symptoms typically last less than 10 minutes, and are usually followed by a unilateral headache. She recalls one visual aura that was followed by right arm numbness and tingling, but this sensory disturbance only lasted a few minutes. In the emergency department, she endorses a throbbing, right-sided headache, which is associated with photophobia, phonophobia, and nausea. At the onset of this episode, she took sumatriptan, which is usually effective, but it did not seem to improve her symptoms. She denies any weakness, numbness/tingling on the left side, difficulty speaking, or difficulty understanding spoken language. Her past medical history is otherwise unremarkable. She has a family history of migraine. She denies tobacco, alcohol, or recreational drug use.

On examination, vital signs are within normal limits. The patient has intact sensation with preserved strength. Extraocular movements were intact, but a dense visual field cut is noted on the right side. The rest of her neurological exam is unremarkable. A non-contrast head CT was negative for acute pathology, however a brain MRI revealed an acute left occipital infarct (Figure 4.1).

What do you do now?

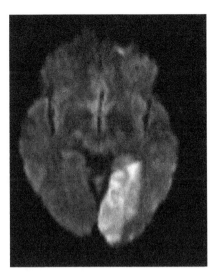

FIGURE 4.1 Diffusion weighted MRI Brain image demonstrating an acute left occipital infarct.

MIGRAINE AND STROKE

It can be easy to dismiss this case as a typical migraine with aura in a young female patient with a prior history of similar episodes, but the persistence of aura beyond 60 minutes should prompt further neurological evaluation. The brain MRI in this patient confirmed an acute stroke, and her diagnosis is highly suspicious for a migrainous infarction. A migraine-induced stroke or migrainous infarction has specific criteria, which have been set by the International Classification of Headache Disorders, Third Beta Edition (ICHD). The patient should have a prior history of migraine with aura, and should have a typical aura lasting longer than 60 minutes, with neuroimaging confirming a stroke in the corresponding region of the brain. The stroke cannot be attributed to any other causal mechanism (Box 4.1).[7] When evaluating a stroke in a young adult, in addition to MR imaging, the following should be performed[9]: head and neck angiography, electrocardiogram, hypercoagulability studies, transesophageal echocardiogram, urine toxicology screen, fasting lipid profile, markers of inflammation (i.e., erythrocyte sedimentation rate/ c-reactive protein [ESR/CRP]), basic metabolic panel, and complete blood count. The patient should also be placed on continuous telemetry.

Studies demonstrate a nearly two-fold increased risk of stroke in patients with migraine. In addition, this risk is higher in younger adults, particularly women under 45 years old, and in those with increased frequency of migraine with aura attacks. The combination of smoking and oral contraceptive use among

> BOX 4.1 **Migrainous Infarction**
>
> Description:
> One or more migraine aura symptoms associated with an ischemic brain
> lesion in the appropriate territory, demonstrated by neuroimaging.
> Diagnostic criteria:
>
> A. A migraine attack fulfilling criteria B and C
> B. Occurring in a patient with Migraine with aura and typical of
>   previous attacks, except that one or more aura symptoms persists
>   for >60 minutes
> C. Neuroimaging demonstrates ischemic infarction in a relevant area
> D. Not better accounted for by another diagnosis.

young females with migraine aura has been shown to increase stroke risk by a factor of approximately 9 when compared with women without migraine.[3] The World Health Organization designates combined hormonal contraceptive use in patients who suffer from migraine with aura as category 4 in terms of medical eligibility criteria. This category states that the condition poses an unacceptable health risk, and that alternative contraceptives should be considered.[8]

Despite these risk factors, migrainous infarction is very infrequent, according to the Lausanne Stroke Registry and the Dijon Stroke Registry, which demonstrated migraine-induced strokes occurring in 0.3% and 0.5% of cases, respectively.[4,5]

The pathophysiology leading to migrainous infarction or to an increased risk of stroke remains unclear, although several theories have been speculated. These include cortical spreading depression (CSD) leading to stroke, increased rate of patent foramen ovale (PFO) in patients with migraine, and the questionable increased risk of cervical artery dissection.

CSD is thought to usually originate in the occipital lobe and to be responsible for migraine aura. CSD is characterized by a wave of neuronal depolarization followed by suppression crossing vascular territories, with related changes in blood flow moving across the cerebral cortex at a rate of 3 mm/min. Some of the changes in blood flow include both hyperemia and transient oligemia, which may lead to migrainous infarction.[2]

The association between migraine and PFO has been demonstrated in a case controlled study performed by Anzola et al. The authors concluded that 48% of patients who suffered from migraine with aura were also found to have a PFO, compared to 23% of patients who have migraine without aura, and 20% in a control group. Given the increased risk of stroke in patients who have migraine with aura and the association of PFO in these migraineurs, the mechanism could potentially be explained by paradoxical emboli.[2]

Regarding cervical artery dissection, a recent meta-analysis concluded that migraine nearly doubled the risk of dissection. The risk was noted to be slightly higher in patients who suffer from migraine with aura, but this was not found to be statistically significant. The etiology of this increased risk still remains uncertain.[3]

Despite evidence suggesting that there is an increased risk of stroke in patients with migraine with aura, the absolute risk of stroke still remains relatively low.

KEY POINTS TO REMEMBER

- Migrainous infarction should be considered in any patient who has a persistent aura lasting longer than 60 minutes.
- There is a two-fold increased risk of stroke in patients with migraine. This is particularly true for women under the age of 45 who suffer from migraine with aura.
- Theories potentially explaining the increase risk of stroke include vascular changes associated with cortical spreading depression, higher rates of patent foramen ovale, and the association with cervical artery dissection.

References

1. Bousser M, Welch KM. Relation between migraine and stroke. *Lancet Neurol.* 2005;4(9):533–542. doi:10.1016/s1474-4422(05)70164-2
2. Katsarava Z, Weimar C. Migraine and stroke. *J Neurol Sci.* 2010;299(1–2):42–44. doi:10.1016/j.jns.2010.08.058
3. Kurth T, Diener H. Migraine and stroke: perspectives for stroke physicians. *Stroke.* 2012;43(12):3421–3426. doi:10.1161/strokeaha.112.656603
4. Milhaud D, Bogousslavsky J, Melle GV, Liot P. Ischemic stroke and active migraine. *Neurology.* 2001;57(10):1805–1811. doi:10.1212/wnl.57.10.1805
5. Sochurkova D, Moreau T, Lemesle M, Menassa M, Giroud M, Dumas R. Migraine history and migraine-induced stroke in the Dijon Stroke Registry. *Neuroepidemiology.* 1999;18(2):85–91. doi:10.1159/000069411
6. Spector JT, Kahn SR, Jones MR, Jayakumar M, Dalal D, Nazarian S. Migraine headache and ischemic stroke risk: an updated meta-analysis. *Am J Med.* 2010;123(7):612–624. doi:10.1016/j.amjmed.2009.12.021
7. The International Classification of Headache Disorders, 3rd ed. (beta version). *Cephalalgia.* 2013;33(9):629–808. doi:10.1177/0333102413485658
8. World Health Organization. 2015. *Medical Eligibility Criteria for Contraceptive Use.* 5th ed. Geneva: World Health Organization, p. 126.
9. Mackey J. Evaluation and management of stroke in young adults. *Continuum.* 2014;20, 352–369. doi:10.1212/01.con.0000446106.74796.e9

5 Seizures Occurring Once a Month

M. Angela O'Neal

A 36-year-old woman is referred for evaluation for epilepsy, which had started one year previously. Her boyfriend, who had witnessed many of the seizures, described them as beginning with a yawn, followed by a high-pitched scream. The patient then would lose tone. This was followed by a tonic posture with arms flexed and legs extended. Occasionally she would then have brief clonic movements. The seizures were usually 1–2 minutes in duration and followed by a postictal confusion lasting up to 15 minutes. She usually has one seizure a month, typically at the onset of her menses. Her menses are regular. She is currently on levetiracetam 500 mg in the morning and 750 mg at night. Brain MRI was normal. Her electroencephalogram was also normal.

Her exam is normal.

What do you do now?

CATAMENIAL EPILEPSY

Hormones can alter seizure frequency, through modulation of brain excitability as well as through their effect on anticonvulsant drug concentrations. Animal studies have suggested that estrogen is a proconvulsant. Whereas progesterone, particularly its metabolite allopregnanolone, promotes neuroinhibition and acts as an anticonvulsant.[1]

Catamenial epilepsy is defined when seizure frequency increases correlated with certain phases of the menstrual cycle. A catamenial pattern may be seen with any type of epilepsy, but it is more common with focal epilepsies. Using the definition that there is a doubling of seizure frequency associated with a particular phase of the menstrual cycle, up to one-third of women have catamenial epilepsy.

A normal menstrual cycle is 28 days, with day 1 defined as the first day of menses, and day 14, the day of ovulation. The first half of the menstrual cycle, days 1–14, is called the *follicular phase*, and the second half, days -14 to -1, the *luteal phase*. Different patterns of catamenial epilepsy have been described. The most common type, as demonstrated by this patient, is the perimenstrual exacerbation, (C1). This corresponds to a progesterone decline. The next most common pattern is the periovulatory exacerbation, (C2). This is characterized by an increase in seizure frequency associated with ovulation and the associated surge in estrogen. The luteal pattern, (C3), is the least frequent. In this pattern, seizure frequency increases in the luteal phase of the menstrual cycle. This is associated with relatively low progesterone levels and anovulatory cycles.[2]

Most treatments have focused on the C1 pattern. Acetozolamide at doses of 250–500 mg daily, three to seven days before menses, has been shown to be efficacious. Benzodiazepines have also been used especially for seizure clusters. The only benzodiazepine proven to have efficacy is clobazem. In a randomized controlled trial, clobazem was shown to be more effective than placebo. A trial with cyclic progesterone lozenges was ineffective in women with intractable partial seizures. However, there was a benefit for the subgroup of women with the C1 pattern who had greater than three times exacerbation of their seizures. The final strategy would be to increase the anticonvulsant dose during the phase of the catamenial exacerbation.[3]

KEY POINTS TO REMEMBER

1. Many women have a catamenial exacerbation of their epilepsy.
2. Defining the specific catamenial pattern is an important step in deciding on treatment strategy.
3. Acetozolamide, clobazem, and cyclic progesterone lozenges, for the C1 pattern only, are effective in suppressing the catamenial seizure exacerbation. An alternative approach would be to increase the antiepileptic drug dose during the time of exacerbation.

References

1. Harden CL, Pennell PB. Neuroendocrine considerations in the treatment of men and women with epilepsy. *Lancet Neurol.* 2013;12(1):72–83.
2. Herzog AG, Klein P, Ransil BJ. Three patterns of catamenial epilepsy. *Epilepsia.* 1997;38:1082–1088.
3. Pennell PB. Pregnancy, epilepsy, and women's issues. *Continuum.* 2013;19(3):697–714.

6 Multiple Ovarian Cysts in a Woman with Epilepsy

M. Angela O'Neal

A 24-year-old woman with idiopathic partial with secondary generalized epilepsy presents to your clinic. Her seizures began at age 12. She experiences no aura; witnesses have reported her seizures to be generalized tonic followed by clonic movements with associated incontinence. She experiences postictal confusion lasting around 30 minutes. Prior brain MRI was normal and previous EEGs have demonstrated a left temporal epileptiform focus. Since age 15, she has been on valproate, with no seizures for two years. She has gained 30 pounds over the last several years.

Her past medical history is remarkable for irregular periods for which she was recently evaluated by an obstetrician gynecologist. Her labs showed an elevated testosterone level, and abdominal ultrasound showed multiple ovarian cysts. A diagnosis of polycystic ovarian syndrome (PCOS) was made.

Her medications are a Mirena IUD and Depakote ER 750 mg bid.

She is 64 inches tall and weighs 225 lbs. Her weight is predominantly central, and she has alopecia in a male pattern. Her neurological exam is normal.

What do you do now?

ANTIEPILEPTIC DRUGS AND POLYCYSTIC OVARIAN SYNDROME

Epilepsy as a Cause of Reproductive Dysfunction

There are numerous reports that epilepsy, particularly focal epilepsy, can cause hypothalamic dysfunction. However, many of these studies are confounded by being retrospective, using subjects who presented to tertiary epilepsy centers and are on treatment with AEDs. There are multiple connections between the limbic cortex and hypothalamus that modulate the hypothalamus–pituitary hormonal secretion. For example, it is well known that, following a generalized seizure, there can be elevated prolactin levels. The gonadotropin-releasing hormone (GnRH) is vulnerable to injury following seizures. Dysfunction of GnRH may lead to abnormal release of follicle-stimulating hormone (FSH) and luteinizing hormone (LH), with direct effects on ovulation and the maturation of ovarian follicles. In addition, there has been some suggestion from small studies that a left temporal focus may be more associated with PCOS.[1]

Polycystic Ovarian Syndrome

PCOS is a diagnosis made on ultrasound and per anatomical criteria, with these showing the presence of multiple ovarian cysts. This is distinct from PCOS where there is endocrine dysfunction. The National Institute of Health consensus definition of PCOS includes the presence of menstrual dysfunction, clinical evidence of hyperandrogenism, and exclusion of other endocrinopathies, such as Cushing's syndrome and hypothyroidism. The etiology of PCOS is felt to be heterogenous, related to a complex interaction between both genetic and environmental factors. PCOS develops when the ovaries are stimulated to produce excessive testosterone. There are several ways this can occur. First, in women who have PCOS, there is to an abnormal pulse frequency and amplitude of LH. The increased levels of LH drive the ovarian thecal cells to produce more androgen. Many women with PCOS have insulin resistance and are obese. This leads to an increased frequency of GnRH pulses and an increase of LH/FSH, causing increased androgen production.

Anti-Epilepsy Drugs and Polycystic Ovarian Syndrome

Valproate is the AED most associated with PCOS. Valproate can directly increase ovarian testosterone production. It can also cause weight gain leading to insulin resistance, another mechanism contributing to PCOS. One study looked at switching women with PCOS from valproate to lamotrigine. In the subsequent year, the women had significant weight loss, decreased androgen levels, and a decrease in the number of ovarian follicles.[2,3]

In our patient, she has had a significant weight gain of 30 lbs., which is probably related to valproate and is contributing to the metabolic syndrome of PCOS. There should be consideration of switching her to another AED, especially as there are additional teratogenic concerns in a woman of childbearing age. Levetiracetam would be a good choice as an AED for this woman.

KEY POINTS TO REMEMBER

1. Epilepsy may contribute to reproductive dysfunction.
2. Women with epilepsy, especially if treated with valproate, are at high risk to develop PCOS.
3. PCOS is a complex disorder with both genetic and environmental contributors. It develops in women where the ovaries are stimulated to produce excessive testosterone.

References

1. Harden C, Pennell P. Neuroendocrine considerations in the treatment of men and women with epilepsy. *Lancet Neurol.* 2013;12:72–83.
2. Bilo L, Meo R. Polycystic ovary syndrome in women using valproate: a review. *Gynecol Endocrinol.* 2008;24(10):562–570.
3. Duncan S. Polycystic ovarian syndrome in women with epilepsy: a review. *Epilepsia.* 2001;42(suppl 3):60–65.

7 Newlywed with Headache, Morning Sickness, and Subjective Right-side Weakness

NaTosha N. Gatson and Terri L. Woodard

A 26-year-old right-handed woman presented to her primary care physician with a two-month history of headaches that are worse upon awakening with increasing episodes of nausea, fatigue, and a sense that she is "not as strong as usual" in her right arm. The patient noted that her symptoms did not initially limit her overall ability to work, but she had noticed a steady progression since onset about two months ago. She had returned from her honeymoon two weeks prior to presentation and had initially attributed her symptoms to "stress" and "poor diet" due to wedding planning. She denied seizures. There had been no changes in vision, speech, mentation, or gait. She underwent a contrasted head CT which was concerning for a left cerebral mass. The patient was sent for brain MRI and referred to the neuro-oncologist for further evaluation and recommendation (Figure 7.1).

On examination by neuro-oncology, her pulse is 108; otherwise vitals are normal, and the patient is visibly anxious. Speech and cognition are normal. She has bilateral papilledema, slight right facial droop, decreased acuity right visual field, decreased strength in right hemi-body proximally and distally to 4+/5 in arm and 5–/5 in the leg, reflexes are normal and symmetrical, and sensation is normal to touch, pin, temperature, and vibration. Remainder of examination is otherwise unremarkable. The neuro-oncologist begins to discuss the most likely diagnosis, and next steps. Overwhelmed, the patient interrupts, "But my husband and I are planning to start a family!"

What do you do now?

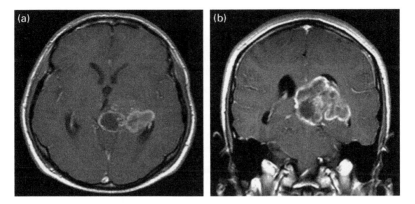

FIGURE 7.1   Magnetic Resonance Imaging (MRI) of brain, T1 weighted post-contrast images. Enhancing lesion of left thalamus on axial (a), and coronal (b) views with noted mass effect on surrounding brain structures.
Photo courtesy of Dr. Steven Toms, Neurosurgeon.

INFERTILITY ASSOCIATED WITH CANCER TREATMENT

Thalamic Glioblastoma, Limited Treatment Options, and Family Planning

Delays in time-to-diagnosis are usually multifactorial. Often, early signs of a developing brain tumor are vague, intermittent, and less likely to alarm patients to seek immediate medical attention. Social, behavioral, or occupational influences, as shown in this case, further hinder patients from seeking medical advice. In addition to patient-related delays to diagnosis, primary care providers sometimes defer ordering brain imaging for such isolated symptoms in a previously healthy patient. More commonly, the patient described in this case would first be ruled out for pregnancy, viral infectious etiology, or even physical/emotional exhaustion. Reports of worsening headache, objective focal weakness, and occupational disability, however, are more ominous, and clinicians are likely to pursue advanced brain imaging. Ultimately, in the above case, the patient was found to have a left-sided deep brain glioblastoma (GBM).

GBM is the most lethal primary brain tumor in adults. Despite decades of research aimed at improving patient outcomes, receiving optimized multimodality treatment (including maximal resection, radiation, and chemotherapy) only offers patients a median overall survival of about 15 months.[1,2] GBM is difficult to treat due to various factors related to the tumor's aggressiveness, paucity of therapies that cross the blood–brain barrier, and often the tumor's location, which limits maximal surgical debulking. In the presented case, the patient has a dominant-side deep brain lesion that presents a major neurosurgical risk for bleeding, severe morbidity, and mortality. Gross total resection is unrealistic in this case, and subtotal resection, radiation, and chemotherapy are the available management options. The patient might also choose no treatment with the understanding that the aggressive tumor will continue to grow, causing disability and ultimately, death. Also important to this case is timely initiation of therapy. These tumors are very aggressive, and treatment delays result in tumor progression and possibly hastened loss of neurological function. However, treatment planning should never supersede the education and desires of the patient as it pertains to treatment.

Use of systemic chemotherapy and radiation to sensitive brain structures could impact patient fertility and should be discussed upfront in this case. The patient should be informed of her risk of treatment-related infertility, and offered referral to a fertility specialist for discussion of fertility preservation (FP) options that may be available. Discussion includes: (1) assessment of baseline fertility and options for FP, (2) issues surrounding pregnancy after cancer, (3) other options for achieving future parenthood, and (4) follow-up throughout her survivorship course as indicated.[3,4]

Issues of survivorship are relevant to address before as well as during the course of treatment. Survivorship-centered practices are often designed to anticipate patient and caregiver needs. These include social work and case-management involvement to address potential medical-legal concerns (power of attorney for healthcare and advance directives), to direct the patient to financial resources (treatment, travel, insurance), and to educate about palliative care and area hospice support.

In summary, delays in diagnosis and initiation of treatment are common hurdles in cancer care. At times, even early diagnosis does not improve our ability to consistently deliver optimal care, due to factors related to tumor location, available therapies, and treatment-related risks. Clinicians must remain mindful of risks associated with the disease as well as treatment of the disease, as these risks might impact the patient, her caregivers, and her overall quality of life (QOL).

KEY POINTS TO REMEMBER

- Treatment: Maximal surgical debulking of tumors is not always a viable option, and patients should understand risks and benefits of the available treatment modalities, including the decision NOT to treat the tumor. Involvement of palliative care teams may be indicated.

- Ethics: Discussions that address fertility preservation, family planning, and pregnancy prevention should be completed and documented prior to initiation of any treatment.
- Survivorship: This usually involves educational, social, and emotional support of patient, which often extends to the caregivers.

References
1. Gilbert MR, Wang M, Aldape KD, et al. Dose-dense temozolomide for newly diagnosed glioblastoma: a randomized phase III clinical trial. *J Clin Oncol.* 2013;31(32):4085–4091.
2. Stupp R, Mason WP, Van Den Bent MJ, et al. 2005. Radiotherapy plus concomitant and adjuvant temozolomide for glioblastoma. *N Engl J Med.* 2005;352(10):987–996.
3. Loren AW, Mangu PB, Beck LN, et al. Fertility preservation for patients with cancer: American Society of Clinical Oncology clinical practice guideline update. *J Clin Oncol.* 2013 Jul 1;31(19):2500–2510.
4. Ethics Committee of the American Society for Reproductive Medicine. Fertility preservation and reproduction in patients facing gonadotoxic therapies: a committee opinion. *Fertil Steril.* 2013;100(5):1224–1231.

8 Routine Long-Term Epilepsy Follow-up

NaTosha N. Gatson

A 28-year-old right-handed woman presents to her neurologist for continued management of her epilepsy condition. She denies having any changes in her seizure frequency, duration, or semiology. She reports her last seizure was 10 months ago (generalized tonic-clonic) due to medication noncompliance and dehydration. The patient is otherwise healthy and without complaints. She has been on her current AED since age nine without any concerns and is tolerating therapy well. During your interview, you obtain a social history, which notes the patient is a graduate student, currently sexually active with a long-term boyfriend, uses oral contraceptives, drinks three to four alcoholic beverages per month on social occasions, drives regularly, and denies use of illicit drugs or tobacco.

Her current medications include a daily vitamin B_{12} supplement and valproic acid (500 mg by mouth three times daily). She reports having recently completed a course of antibiotics for a complicated urinary tract infection earlier in the month. Her examination is normal. A urine pregnancy test completed during clinic visit was *positive*.

What do you do now?

TERATOGENIC MEDICATION

Unplanned Pregnancy, AED Choice, and Teratogenicity Risk Factors

The case described has several classic concerns that could have been addressed at various time points throughout the physician–patient relationship.

Epilepsy is the third most common chronic neurological disorder worldwide. Unfortunately, all first-line therapies used to treat seizure are associated with some level of risk to the fetus *in utero*. The U.S. Food and Drug Administration recently published the "Pregnancy and Lactation Labeling Rule," which changes the format of prescription drug packaging inserts. Specifically, in the pregnancy subsection, former A, B, C, D, X lettering categories used to designate pregnancy risk were replaced with information including a summary of risks, available data, and clinical considerations. These changes aim to better assist providers with evaluating risks versus benefits for using medications in pregnant or nursing mothers (FDA Pregnancy and Lactation Labeling (Drugs) Final Rule, 2014 [accessed Oct. 19, 2016]. Available from: http://www.fda.gov/Drugs/DevelopmentApprovalProcess/DevelopmentResources/Labeling/ucm093307.htm).

Despite decades of research in the area, few mechanism-targeted therapeutics to treat seizures are available. Instead, patients with epilepsy are treated symptomatically. For this and other reasons, understanding the biological triggers and susceptibilities for seizures is paramount. Interestingly, there are known bidirectional influences of epileptic events on hormonal activity in the central nervous system (CNS). Outside of the role for sex hormones on reproductive and neuronal tissues—epileptic events themselves have been demonstrated to modulate hormone levels.[1] In the above case, as the patient came of a reproductive age, the clinician might have reconsidered the anti-epileptic therapy being used, based on frequency of dosing and risk in reproductive-aged women. With recent advances in the field, the decision to use a medication with a better safety profile, such as levetiracetam, usually dosed twice daily, should be considered. While it is notable that all AEDs have some risk for teratogenicity, after the first trimester of pregnancy, the actual seizure event has been reported to increase fetal morbidity and risk pregnancy maintenance. These risks include fetal trauma related to falls, fetal heart rate deceleration, placental abruption, miscarriage, preterm labor, or premature birth.[2]

In the United States, between 40% and 60% of pregnancies are either unplanned or unintended. In a recently reported retrospective study of 115 women on teratogenic medications, nearly 70% were not using concurrent medical contraception. For the nearly 30% using contraception, oral contraceptives (OCs) had been the method of choice. Sadly, less than 7% reported receiving any counseling for a contraceptive plan.[3] In the above case, it would have been appropriate to discuss the potential for drug–drug interactions in a patient on OCs and AEDs. The patient could have potentially experienced failure of her OC and/or her AED secondary to a drug–drug interaction with use of an antibiotic regimen while on therapy.

A discussion about future pregnancy planning is appropriate at the first visit and at several points throughout the physician–patient relationship to cover treatment regimens and potential associated risks. Once a pregnancy has been diagnosed in a patient with epilepsy, it is important to link the patient with the appropriate obstetric providers to best evaluate the fetus over the course of the pregnancy, as well as offer more education to the parents. Considering the patient's wishes to continue or terminate the pregnancy might also present a need for referral to outside appropriate providers. This case is a challenge because the patient is now known to be pregnant while on AEDs and OCs, and there is a potential for other medication and substance exposure to the fetus based on the clinical history provided. Fetal or pregnancy complications might be multifactorial.[4,5]

KEY POINTS TO REMEMBER

- Prevention: Consider modification of AED of choice in reproductive-aged women.
- Prevention: Folic acid supplementation prior to pregnancy has been shown to significantly reduce the risk for neural tube defects.
- Prevention: Frequently discuss pregnancy planning, pregnancy prevention, and common drug–drug interactions in all patients on therapy.
- Evaluation: Always order a pregnancy test for patients with reasonable risk factors prior to prescribing high-risk teratogenic therapies.
- Ethics and referral: Make referral for fertility and reproductive health assessment and education for patients with high risk pregnancy.

References

1. Velíšková J, Desantis KA. Sex and hormonal influences on seizures and epilepsy. *Horm Behav.* 2013 Feb;63(2):267–277.
2. Kaplan PW, Norwitz ER, Ben-Menachem E, et al. Obstetric risks for women with epilepsy during pregnancy. *Epilepsy Behav.* 2007 Nov;11(3):283–291.

3. Bhakta J, Bainbridge J, Borgelt L. Teratogenic medications and concurrent contraceptive use and women of childbearing ability with epilepsy. *Epilepsy Behav*. 2015 Nov;52(PtA):212–217.

4. Borgelt LM, Hart FM, Bainbridge JL. Epilepsy during pregnancy: focus on management strategies. *Int J Womens Health*. 2016 Sep 19;8:505–517. eCollection 2016.

5. Bauer J, Isojarvi JI, Herzog AG, et al. Reproductive dysfunction in women with epilepsy: recommendations for evaluation and management. *J Neurol Neurosurg Psychiatry*. 2002;73:121–125.

9 A Young Woman with Infertility

Alexandra Lovett and Whitney W. Woodmansee

A 28-year-old female presents with infertility. Menarche developed at age 17, and she was diagnosed with PCOS at age 18. Menses had been irregular and she was started on oral contraceptives. These were continued for 10 years. When pregnancy was desired, oral contraceptives were discontinued. Menses did not resume.

On review of systems, she reported a long history of headaches, which were assumed to be migraines. They occurred approximately once per week and were characterized as right-sided with associated nausea and photophobia. She also reported intermittent galactorrhea with expression over the last three to four years. Her physical examination was normal.

What do you do now?

PROLACTINOMA

Prolactinomas are generally benign and are the most common type of hormone-secreting pituitary adenoma. Most prolactinomas are considered microadenomas, which are defined by size less than 1 centimeter (cm).[1] Macroadenomas (size ≥1 cm) are more likely to cause symptoms associated with mass effect, including but not limited to headaches, cranial nerve abnormalities, and visual disturbances. Classic visual disturbance would be a bitemporal hemianopia due to compression of the optic chiasm; however, patients may have a unilateral hemianopia or quadrantopia depending on where the visual pathway is affected. Hyperprolactinemia is associated with hypogonadotropic hypogonadism, and women may present with galactorrhea, menstrual irregularities, and infertility; however, many women are asymptomatic. Postmenopausal women and men with prolactinomas tend to present later with larger tumors and accompanying mass effects than premenopausal women, since there is no observable disruption of a menstrual cycle in these individuals.

In assessing a woman with infertility, serum prolactin levels should always be checked. In most laboratory assays, a prolactin level of less than 25 micrograms/liter (μg/L) would be considered normal for a nonpregnant woman.[1,2] Prolactin levels of greater than 10 times the laboratory upper limit of normal[3] or greater than 250 μg/L are often considered diagnostic of a prolactinoma.[4,5] If the prolactin level is elevated, a thorough investigation of potential etiologies should be performed to assess for physiological and medication-induced causes. A pregnancy test and TSH level should be checked, as both pregnancy and primary hypothyroidism can cause hyperprolactinemia.[2-4] The patient's medication list should be reviewed for medications that are associated with hyperprolactinemia, with the most common culprits being dopamine antagonist medications, including but not limited to antipsychotics, antihistamines, antidepressants, estrogen agonists, cholinergic agonists, and antiemetics.[2-4] Of note, exercise, sleep, stress, and breastfeeding can cause a physiological hyperprolactinemia.[2-4] Chronic renal and hepatic failure can reduce the clearance of prolactin and cause hyperprolactinemia.[2-4] If the patient is not pregnant, and the above factors are excluded, an elevated prolactin level should then prompt an MRI study with a pituitary protocol, which would entail thin coronal sections through the pituitary and the administration of intravenous (IV) gadolinium. The normal pituitary gland is homogenously enhancing and fits nicely into the sella turcica, with a rounded appearance. The upper portion of the pituitary is usually flat or convex in shape; the infundibulum can be appreciated, as well as the optic chiasm superiorly. An adenoma is usually a hypoenhancing mass within the pituitary gland itself (see Figure 9.1). If it is not contained within

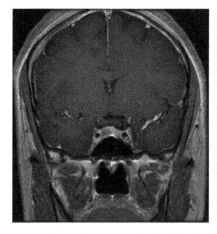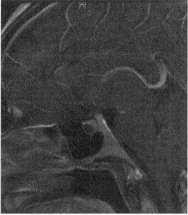

FIGURE 9.1 Magnetic resonance imaging (MRI) of the brain in coronal (*left*) and sagittal (*right*) sections with IV contrast. A hypoenhancing pituitary adenoma is visible adjacent to the right internal carotid artery (ICA).

the gland and rises above the sella, it is often a macroadenoma. If it approaches the optic chiasm in size, formal Humphrey visual fields should be assessed and trended in follow-up. Any suprasellar tumor, such as a nonfunctioning pituitary adenoma or craniopharyngioma, can cause hyperprolactinemia due to what is termed "stalk effect." The mechanism for this is via compression of the infundibular stalk, which prevents dopamine-induced inhibition of prolactin secretion or impaired production of dopamine by the hypothalamus.[2] If the MRI is consistent with a macroadenoma and the prolactin is only mildly elevated (<200 μg/L), a repeat prolactin level with dilution should be obtained to rule out the "hook effect" that can occur in some prolactin assays and lead to a false underestimation of very high prolactin levels.[2,4,5]

Once a prolactinoma is diagnosed, treatment should be considered based on the individual patient's assessment. Asymptomatic patients with microadenomas do not necessarily warrant treatment other than observation.[4,5] Estrogen replacement therapy can also be used to restore menses in women with microprolactinomas not seeking fertility.[4,5] For patients with symptomatic microadenomas and most macroadenomas, the initial treatment of choice is pharmacological, with dopamine agonist therapy with either cabergoline or bromocriptine.[4,5] Cabergoline is generally the preferred dopamine agonist due to its superior tolerability and efficacy. However, in this patient, who wishes to become pregnant, bromocriptine should be used over cabergoline as it has a longer safety record in pregnancy, with long-term studies showing no increased risk of miscarriage or negative effects on the fetus.[1,4–6] Once pregnancy is confirmed, it is recommended that dopamine agonist therapy be discontinued.[4-6] Since pregnancy is associated with lactotroph hyperplasia, prolactinoma patients must be followed very closely during pregnancy for signs of tumor progression and counseled on red-flag symptoms, including but not limited to sudden-onset or progressive headache, neck stiffness, visual field loss, or double vision. Patients are followed clinically and not with scheduled MRI or prolactin levels during pregnancy. Patients with macroadenomas are typically at higher risk of mass effects (i.e., visual loss) from tumor enlargement, and visual field testing is recommended every two to three months during pregnancy.[4-6] New symptoms could indicate either adenoma enlargement or pituitary apoplexy and should prompt an urgent pituitary MRI without gadolinium and consideration for reinitiation of bromocriptine if tumor progression occurs.[4-6]

In general, medical therapy for prolactinomas should be trialed first, even in macroadenoma patients with visual loss due to chiasmal compression.[4,5] Failure of dopamine agonist (DA) treatment is marked by inability to achieve a normal prolactin level and a 50% reduction in tumor size with maximal medical therapy.[4,5] Neurosurgical tumor resection is typically reserved for patients who are intolerant of or resistant to DA therapy, and radiation therapy should be reserved for resistant or malignant prolactinomas.[4,5]

Prolactinoma patients require long-term monitoring of prolactin levels, tumor status, and general pituitary function. Prolactin levels often correlate with tumor size and tumor expansion and should be monitored initially every three months for the first year (when the risk of recurrence is highest), and then yearly in stable patients with significant increases or symptoms prompting an MRI.[1,4] Although recurrence rates are high, DA therapy can be discontinued in some patients who have had a documented response and clinical stability.[4,5]

KEY POINTS TO REMEMBER

- In the female patient with infertility and hyperprolactinemia, pregnancy, primary hypothyroidism and medication-induced process must be ruled out. If no other etiology is identified, a pituitary MRI should be performed to identify a prolactin-producing pituitary adenoma.
- Medical therapy with a dopamine agonist is the treatment of choice for most prolactinomas. Cabergoline is the preferred agent due to better tolerability and efficacy, but bromocriptine is often used if

pregnancy is desired. Small asymptomatic prolactinomas can be followed conservatively.

. Dopamine agonist therapy should be stopped when pregnancy is confirmed. Patients should be followed clinically for signs of enlarging prolactinoma (headaches, visual field deficits) or pituitary apoplexy during the remainder of the pregnancy.

References

1. Almalki MH, Alzahrani S, Alshahrani F, et al. Managing prolactinomas during pregnancy. *Front Endocrinol (Lausanne)*. 2015;6:85.
2. Cortet-Rudelli C, Sapin R, Bonneville JF, et al. Etiological diagnosis of hyperprolactinemia. *Ann Endocrinol (Paris)*. 2007;68:98–105.
3. Klibanski A. Prolactinomas. *N Engl J Med*. 2010;362:1219–1226.
4. Melmed S, Casanueva FF, Hoffman AR, et al. Diagnosis and treatment of hyperprolactinemia: an Endocrine Society clinical practice guideline. *J Clin Endocrinol Metab*. 2011;96:273–288.
5. Schlechte JA. Long-term management of prolactinomas. *J Clin Endocrinol Metab*. 2007;92:2861–2865.
6. Wong A, Anderson Eloy J, Couldwell WT, Liu JK. Update on prolactinomas. Part 1: clinical manifestations and diagnostic challenges. *J Clin Neurosci*. 2015;22:1562–1567.

10 A Woman with Weight Gain and Fatigue

Alexandra Lovett and
Whitney W. Woodmansee

A 38-year-old woman with hypothyroidism sustained a left humerus fracture and underwent an open reduction and internal fixation (ORIF). On review of systems, she reported 10 years of weight gain with a current body mass index (BMI) of 39. Over the last three to four years, she developed headaches, fatigue, and hirsutism. Her menses were regular. She was diagnosed with hypertension, diabetes mellitus type II, and osteopenia. On examination she had a round face and was obese. She had purple striae, dorsocervical and supraclavicular fat, facial hirsutism, and a healing fracture. Neurological examination was unremarkable.

What do you do now?

CUSHING'S DISEASE

Cushing's disease is hypercortisolemia that is pituitary-dependent, as opposed to Cushing's syndrome from an adrenal lesion, an ectopic tumor secreting adrenocorticotropic hormone (ACTH) or corticotrophin-releasing hormone (CRH), or exogenous corticosteroids.[1] In Cushing's disease, there is typically an ACTH-secreting pituitary adenoma, which then acts on the adrenal gland to produce cortisol, which additionally causes a negative feedback loop to suppress the secretion of CRH from the hypothalamus and disrupt the hypothalamic-pituitary-adrenal (HPA) axis.[1] The pituitary adenoma, in this case, is often a microadenoma as opposed to a macroadenoma with a lower likelihood of signs of mass effect (see the chapter on prolactinoma).[1,2] Cushing's disease is at least three times more prevalent in women than in men and is usually diagnosed in the fourth to sixth decades of life.[1]

Clinically, patients with Cushing's syndrome, either from ectopic tumors, exogenous steroids, or pituitary adenomas, will present similarly. Symptoms will include weight gain, fatigue, easy bruising, and increased hair growth.[1,2] Objectively on physical examination, patients are often overweight or obese but may have a Cushingoid appearance in terms of fat distribution. There is often a "buffalo hump" with adipose deposition over the neck as well as abdominal fat deposition. The extremities are thinner, and patients will have "moon facies" with a circular appearance to the face. Skin changes can include acne, purple striae, and acanthosis nigricans, which is thick dark skin often seen in the axilla and other skin folds. Patients with Cushing's syndrome may have multiple comorbidities, including but not limited to diabetes mellitus, hypertension, hyperlipidemia, osteoporosis, infertility, immunosuppression leading to an elevated risk of infection, and neuropsychiatric disorders including depression and anxiety; these comorbidities can often lead to mortality in patients with Cushing's disease.[1,2]

In regards to effects on the nervous system from Cushing's disease, patients are often myopathic with proximal muscle weakness on examination. There is often neurocognitive impairment with memory difficulties predominating, but additionally with impaired language performance and verbal learning being documented as well.[1]

Once there is clinical suspicion for Cushing's disease, further testing should be sought to achieve the diagnosis, which can be difficult to obtain. Initially, one should look for elevated levels of cortisol by performing a 24-hour urine collection for urinary free cortisol, with normal values being less than 90 micrograms (μg) in 24 hours and levels greater than 300 μg in 24 hours being diagnostic.[2] This test has both a sensitivity and specificity greater than 90%.[2]

Another option in patients who may have difficulty doing a 24-hour urine collection would be a 1 milligram (mg) dexamethasone-suppression test in which the patient would orally take 1 mg of oral dexamethasone at 11:00 pm and have their plasma cortisol measured at 8:00 am the following morning; normal value is less than or equal to 5 µg per deciliter (dl).[2] This test has a 98% sensitivity but a slightly lower specificity of 80%.[2] If both tests are negative, Cushing's disease is unlikely, though testing should be repeated if clinical suspicion remains high.[2] The urinary collection test can also be used to confirm the dexamethasone suppression test.[2]

After confirming Cushing's syndrome with these tests, you must determine if the process is ACTH-dependent or -independent. One method is by measuring a late-afternoon ACTH level (after 4:00 pm).[2] A value greater than 5 picograms per ml (pg/ml) confirms an ACTH-dependent process.[2] Another option is a CRH-stimulation test in which the patient is given 1 µg per kilogram (kg) of intravenous CRH, and levels of ACTH and cortisol are measured before the administration and at multiple time intervals afterward, up to two hours after the injection.[2] If the cortisol level increases by 20% or more above basal level, or the ACTH level increases by 50% or more above basal level, this additionally confirms an ACTH-dependent lesion.[2] Magnetic resonance imaging with pituitary protocol should then be performed to look for an adenoma (see the prolactinoma chapter). If the MRI is unrevealing, inferior petrosal sinus sampling (IPSS) should be performed; this is a catheter-based approach in which ACTH is measured simultaneously from the blood and from the inferior petrosal sinus at one and five minutes.[2,3] CRH is then administered peripherally, and samples of ACTH are again taken from the peripheral vein and the inferior petrosal sinus at specified time intervals.[3] A ratio of 2:1 of petrosal sinus ACTH to peripheral ACTH at baseline, or a ratio of 3:1 after CRH administration, would confirm a pituitary source of ACTH production and can also help determine the side of the adenoma, whether left or right, for surgical planning.[2,3]

Once a pituitary adenoma has been found, neurosurgical intervention via transsphenoidal resection of the adenoma is indicated.[1,2] Patients may then become deficient in cortisol and require exogenous replacement with steroids in the perioperative period; however, hormone levels should be trended months after surgery, as lifelong steroids may be required.[2] Recurrence is common, and repeat resection or pituitary irradiation may be necessary.[2] Panhypopituitarism may also be an unintended consequence of pituitary surgery; therefore, all HPA-axis hormone levels should be followed perioperatively and postoperatively, especially cortisol, thyroid-stimulating hormone (TSH), and thyroxine (T4) levels.

- Cushing's disease is pituitary-dependent, as opposed to Cushing's syndrome, which is from either exogenous steroids or ectopic ACTH- or CRH-secreting lesions.
- Cushing's disease can be difficult to diagnose, though multiple methods exist, including 24-hour urinary cortisol-excretion and dexamethasone-suppression testing as initial screens. MRI brain with pituitary protocol and/or IPSS sampling can help localize this process to the pituitary, which increases the likelihood of a diagnosis of Cushing's disease.
- As opposed to treatment of prolactinoma with observation or medical therapy, ACTH-secreting pituitary adenomas are best treated with surgical resection.

References

1. Pivonello R, De Leo M, Cozzolino A, Colao A. (2015) The treatment of Cushing's disease. *Endocr Rev.* 2015;36(4):385–486.
2. Kirk LF Jr., Hash RB, Katner HP, Jones T. Cushing's disease: clinical manifestations and diagnostic evaluation. *Am Fam Physician.* 2000;62:1119–1127.
3. Oldfield EH, Doppman JL, Nieman LK, et al. Petrosal sinus sampling with and without corticotropin-releasing hormone for the differential diagnosis of Cushing's syndrome. *N Engl J Med.* 1991;325:897–905.

11 A 27-Year-Old Woman with Epilepsy Planning for Pregnancy

P. Emanuela Voinescu

A 27-year-old woman with idiopathic generalized epilepsy (IGE), seizure-free for five years on valproic acid (VPA) and levetiracetam (LEV) dual therapy, presents to the epilepsy clinic for preconception counseling. She failed topiramate (TPM) in the past, reportedly had a rash to lamotrigine (LTG), and also failed LEV monotherapy. The epileptologist advises her to start taking folic acid and a prenatal vitamin as soon as possible. He strongly recommends to discontinue VPA and re-attempt LEV monotherapy. This change leads to severe depression, and she is then switched from LEV to LTG. She tolerates the transition fine and she remains seizure-free for three months on LTG monotherapy with stable mood and no recurrent rash. The LTG level after three months on target dose is 4.0 mcg/mL.

An ED physician calls the epileptologist six months later to inform them that the patient had a seizure and that her labs revealed an LTG level of 2.6 mcg/mL and a positive pregnancy test.

What do you do now?

This patient is a woman of childbearing age who carries a diagnosis of epilepsy and is on an antiepileptic medication. The initial therapy, VPA, is known to be highly teratogenic and to have poor neurodevelopmental outcomes, thus she is transitioned to antiepileptic drugs (AEDs) with better profiles during pregnancy, LEV and LTG. Importantly, the LTG level needs close monitoring during pregnancy, when a dramatic decrease in the level may occur, leading to breakthrough seizures.

About 40% of pregnancies in the United States are unplanned, and this percentage is likely to be higher for women with epilepsy (WWE) of childbearing age. This is important information to remember when treating this population, who are on continuous treatment with known teratogens. Organogenesis occurs within the first 4–10 weeks of gestation (post-conception), and structural abnormalities established during this window will be irreversible. Therefore, pregnancy planning should be a topic of discussion for any WWE of childbearing age, ideally prior to pregnancy. However, even if this time window is missed, there are antiepileptic drugs (AEDs) known to further impact the child's neurodevelopment and, potentially, neonatal/obstetrical outcomes. Therefore, optimizing the AED regimen is something that needs to be considered even during pregnancy. In addition, given strong evidence for the beneficial effect of folic acid early in pregnancy, as well as no significant side effects or interaction with other medications, all WWE of childbearing age should be encouraged to take supplemental folic acid.[1]

This patient's regimen is highly problematic: she is on polytherapy, and one of the AEDs is VPA. The 2009 American Academy of Neurology/ American Epilepsy Society practice parameters concluded that polytherapy is associated with a higher risk for major congenital malformations (MCM) as compared to monotherapy, and, while more recent studies challenge this paradigm for some AED combinations, they confirm this to be true for combinations that include VPA. Moreover, it has been repeatedly shown that VPA has the highest rate of MCM, worse neonatal outcomes (high rate for small for gestational age, reduced Apgar scores) and, importantly, impaired neurodevelopment with potential long-lived cognitive disabilities.[2] Therefore, it seems reasonable to attempt discontinuation of VPA as the first step in optimizing this patient's regimen. One needs to be mindful, however, that there are minimal data regarding the safety of altering the AED regimen once seizure freedom has been achieved.

Based on clinical evidence so far, LEV and LTG seem to have the safest profile for MCM risk, and neonatal and neurodevelopmental outcomes.[2] Fortunately, both of these medications are good choices both for IGE, as well as for focal epilepsies. Unfortunately, for IGE, if these medications are not an option, the alternatives have either a significantly inferior safety profile during pregnancy, such as TPM and VPA, or still-insufficient data on their use during pregnancy, such as zonisamide or perampanel. Therefore, it seemed reasonable to reattempt LEV monotherapy for our patient, now seizure-free for five years on dual therapy. Once this failed, it was also reasonable to retry LTG, given that there are frequent symptomatic complaints quickly attributed to an AED, without always considering alternative explanations and sometimes even without objective data. Therefore, for both the patient's well-being (given concern of mood instability) and future pregnancy (given poor VPA profile and excellent LTG profile during pregnancy), the optimal therapy was achieved.

Why did our patient have a seizure, then, and was this preventable? Pregnancy is a special state in which physiological changes can alter the natural course of diseases and change the pharmacokinetics of medications, making the therapeutic management more complicated. In our case, one should first think of LTG pharmacokinetics during pregnancy. LTG is 55% protein-bound and undergoes liver metabolism by uridine 5'-diphospho-glucuronosyltransferase (UGT) enzymes. It is hypothesized that the rising levels of estrogens during pregnancy may induce the UGT enzyme system and consequently increase the metabolism of LTG, leading to decreases in LTG concentrations. It was rigorously proven that, during pregnancy, approximately a quarter of WWE experienced a minimal increase in clearance, while the remaining three-quarters experienced a greater than threefold increase in clearance.[3] In addition, the same authors reported that seizure frequency significantly increased when the LTG level decreased to 65% of the preconception level; this held true for other AEDs as well.[4] These studies emphasize the need to monitor LTG (as well as other AEDs: LTG, VPA, oxcarbazepine) levels during pregnancy.

Our scenario reveals a 65% drop in the presumed steady LTG level, probably explained by pharmacokinetic changes triggered by the new pregnancy and probably the trigger for the breakthrough seizure. This is unlikely to be LTG failure, given six months of seizure freedom, and it might have been preventable if the patient had been instructed to inform her physician about her pregnancy as soon as possible. In addition, although research to date has revealed no overall seizure frequency variation during pregnancy, a significant fraction of women (up to ~25%) may experience some variability during pregnancy, yet data are insufficient to determine what factors are important for this variability.

Once an AED therapy had been chosen as part of preconception planning, experts recommend three practical principles:

1. The dose should be lowered if possible (given evidence that, in addition to the type of AED, dose at conception also affects the rate of MCMs), and this should be especially considered upon the discontinuation of estrogen-containing contraceptive hormones (which lower the levels of several AEDs).
2. A pregnancy individualized target concentration should be established and aimed for slightly higher values when compared to preconception levels (given anticipation for levels dropping as pregnancy progresses, and knowledge that if the levels reach less than 65%, there is a significantly increased risk for breakthrough seizures).
3. Monthly AED levels should be tested and dose readjusted to aim for an individualized target concentration.[5]

Regarding observations about pregnancy-related variability in seizure frequency, seizure freedom rate during pregnancy seems to be higher in WWE with IGE (73.6%) than in those with localization-related epilepsy (59.5%). Also, seizure control prior to pregnancy is the best predictor for seizure control during pregnancy: approximately 90% of WWE remain seizure-free during pregnancy if seizure-free for at least nine months to one year prior to pregnancy, while WWE who had seizures in the pre-pregnancy month had 15-times higher risk for seizures during pregnancy.

KEY POINTS TO REMEMBER

- About 40% of pregnancies in the United States are unplanned, so physicians should proactively educate WWE regarding folate use and AED use during pregnancy.
- Evidence so far discourages the use of valproic acid, as it is the AED with the highest MCM rates and detrimental impact on long-term neurodevelopment, and has found levetiracetam and lamotrigine to be the safest.
- Polytherapy is considered inferior to monotherapy, especially if VPA is one of the agents used.
- Pharmacokinetics knowledge is crucial for managing WWE during pregnancy, and levels need to be checked frequently for most AEDs.

- Practice advice: 1. Lowest AED dose possible; 2. Individualized target AED levels, slightly higher than preconception levels; 3. Monthly level checks during pregnancy.
- Good predictors for seizure control during pregnancy are: genetic generalized epilepsy and seizure freedom nine months prior to pregnancy.

References

1. Harden, Pennell, Koppel, et al. Practice Parameter update: Management issues for women with epilepsy—Focus on pregnancy (an evidence-based review): Vitamin K, folic acid, blood levels, and breastfeeding Report of the Quality Standards Subcommittee and Therapeutics and Technology Assessment Subcommittee of the American Academy of Neurology and American Epilepsy Society. *Neurology*. 2009;73(2):142–149. doi:10.1212/wnl.0b013e3181a6b325.

2. Voinescu PE, Pennell PB. Management of epilepsy during pregnancy. *Expert Rev Neurother*. 2015;15(10):1171–87. doi:10.1586/14737175.2015.1083422.

3. Polepally A, Pennell P, Brundage R, et al. Model-based lamotrigine clearance changes during pregnancy: clinical implication. *Annals of Clinical and Translational Neurology*. 2014;1(2):99–106. doi:10.1002/acn3.29.

4. Reisinger, Newman, Loring, Pennell, Meador. Antiepileptic drug clearance and seizure frequency during pregnancy in women with epilepsy. *Epilepsy & Behavior*. 2013;29(1):13–8. doi:10.1016/j.yebeh.2013.06.026.

5. Pennell P. Use of Antiepileptic Drugs During Pregnancy: Evolving Concepts. *Neurotherapeutics*. 2016. doi:10.1007/s13311-016-0464-0.

Pregnancy

12 What Imaging Test Do I Order?

M. Angela O'Neal

A 28-year-old woman G1P0 (G = *gravid*, the number
of times a woman has been pregnant; P = *partum*, the
number of children to which a woman has given birth),
10 weeks pregnant, was texting her husband when he
noticed her reply made no sense. He called her, and she
seemed very confused. He arrived home 10 minutes later.
When he found her, she was confused, speaking gibberish
with a right facial droop. He called the emergency
medical technicians, who brought her to the emergency
department.

On examination: Her vitals were: blood pressure 140/82,
pulse 78 and regular. She was afebrile. Her language was
fluent with multiple paraphasic errors. She could follow
only one-step commands. She had a left gaze preference,
a right facial droop, and a right arm drift. Her right toe was
upgoing.

What do you do now?

IMAGING DURING PREGNANCY

Our patient most likely has a left middle cerebral infarct. She needs an imaging study in order to decide the appropriate next steps. Our options are either a head computed tomography (CT), or a brain MRI.

Basics of Radiation

A *rad* is the amount of energy deposited per kilogram of tissue, which reflects the absorbed dose of radiation. In the United States, an average person has a whole-body exposure per year to 3.1 rads. Diagnostic imaging procedures typically expose the fetus to less than 5 rads. The effects of radiation are divided into either deterministic, dose-related, or stochastic types, where exposure determines the probability of an outcome. Deterministic effects have a threshold below which the effect does not occur. The threshold may be very small and may vary from person to person. However, once the threshold has been exceeded, the severity of an effect increases with dose; an example is hair loss, which occurs at exposures of 2–5 gray (0.1 rad = 0.01 gray; see Figures 12.1 and 12.2).

Stochastic effects occur by chance and may occur without a threshold level of dose, whose probability is proportional to the dose and whose severity is independent of the dose. In the context of radiation, cancer induction as a result of exposure to radiation occurs in a stochastic manner: there is no threshold point, and risk increases with dose, the severity of the effects do not; the patient will either develop cancer or they will not. (See Figure 12.3)

The amount of radiation exposure to the fetus from a non-contract maternal head CT is 200 mrad (millirads). This is several orders of magnitude less than the

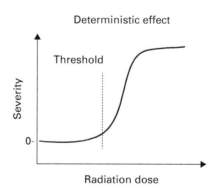

FIGURE 12.1 This graph demonstrates what occurs with deterministic effects. There is a threshold below which an effect does not occur. The threshold level may be different between different populations. For example, the radiation threshold to cause injury is less for an infant as compared with an adult.

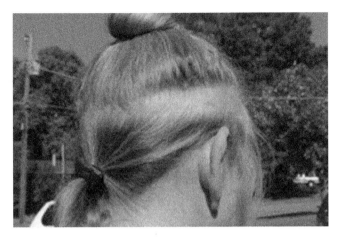

FIGURE 12.2 Hair loss due to radiation is a deterministic effect.

doses of radiation needed to cause fetal loss, growth restriction, or fetal anomalies.[1] However, there is still a risk of a stochastic effect. For this reason, MRI is preferred over CT in pregnancy.[2]

Magnetic Resonance Imaging

MRI has possible biological effects on local electrical fields and related to local heating of tissue. There have been no reported harmful effects from MR imaging in pregnant women. Safety studies have usually used magnets of 1.5 tesla or less. As there is no exposure to ionizing radiation, MRI is the preferred imaging

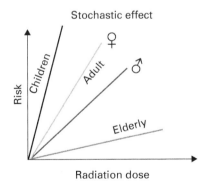

FIGURE 12.3 This figure demonstrates what occurs in a stochastic effect. There is no threshold below which there is no effect. The probability that an effect occurs increases in proportion to the exposure dose, but the severity of the effect is not dose-dependent. Cancer related to radiation exposure is an example.

modality in pregnancy. When possible, it is recommended to postpone a MRI until the second trimester. Gadolinium does cross through the placental barrier and is excreted by the fetus. Due to concerns regarding renal injury to the fetus, gadolinium is avoided when possible.[3]

Imaging in an Emergency

Our patient most likely has had a stroke. This is a neurological emergency. Therefore, a non-contrast head CT is the preferred imaging. The benefit to knowing what is going on in order to plan appropriate therapy clearly outweighs the potential risk of ionizing radiation. In this case, the health of the mother is paramount and will directly determine fetal viability. The treatment should be guided by the stroke characteristics rather than the obstetrical concerns.

KEY POINTS TO REMEMBER

1. The amount of ionizing radiation from most diagnostic imaging procedures is many orders of magnitude less than that needed to cause dose-related, deterministic effects.
2. However, ionizing radiation still has stochastic effects.
3. MRI is the preferred imaging modality in pregnancy.
4. In an emergency, the best imaging is that which can answer the question quickly, as the mother's health is the priority.

References
1. McCollough CH, Schueler BA, Atwell TD, et al. Radiation exposure and pregnancy: when should we be concerned? *Radiographics*. 2007;27:909–917.
2. Austin LM, Frush DP. Compendium of national guidelines for imaging the pregnant patient. *AJR Am J Roentgenol*. 2011;197:W737–W746.
3. De Wilde JP, Rivers AW, Price DL. A review of the current use of magnetic resonance imaging in pregnancy and safety implications for the fetus. *Prog Biophys Mol Biol*. 2005;87:335–353.

13 A Lady with a Headache in the First Trimester

M. Angela O'Neal

A 23-year-old woman who has migraine without aura
is eight weeks pregnant. Her migraines had been well
controlled with sumatriptan. She is now having her usual
headaches with nausea and vomiting several
times a week.

What do you do now?

MIGRAINE

Natural History

Migraines occur three times more frequently in women due to hormonal influences. Menstrual exacerbation of headache is most commonly associated with migraine without aura. In pregnancy, due to changes in the level of estrogen, migraines are often more frequent in the first trimester. Particularly in women who have migraine without aura, 70–80% experience remission by the second trimester.[1,2] Patients who have migraine with aura have a less predictable course during pregnancy, as these headaches are generally less hormonally triggered. Migraineurs have a higher risk of developing eclampsia.[3]

General Strategy

Given that migraine is both a benign disorder, and the natural history that the headaches will go into remission by the second trimester, prophylactic therapy is not generally utilized. In addition, use of prophylactic medications have a risk of teratogenicity and usually take at least four to six weeks to establish efficacy. Therefore, it is recommended to use medications at the time of the migraine attack only. Alternative therapies to minimize migraine triggers, such as stress management and acupuncture, are helpful alternatives to medication.

The pregnancy classification both for medications used for acute migraine and for migraine prevention are shown in Tables 13.1 and 13.2. In the patient who presents to the emergency room with migraine, one proposed strategy for treatment is suggested here. Intravenous (IV) fluids and IV magnesium are safe and effective treatments for migraine in pregnancy (Box 13.1). In refractory patients, the addition of steroids is reasonable. There is significant amount of data around the use of sumatriptan in pregnancy. No major congenital malformations have been identified in large retrospective trials. In the Norwegian registry, use of sumatriptan in the last trimester was associated with a small increase of bleeding during delivery related to uterine atony.[4]

Migraine Management Postpartum

Postpartum, due to sleep deprivation, stress, as well as hormonal fluctuation, migraine frequency often increases. Unlike in pregnancy, there is little risk with use of nonsteroidal anti-inflammatory agents, and triptans are also safe. In addition, if needed, there are multiple safe choices for preventative therapy (Tables 13.1 and 13.2).[5]

TABLE 13.1 **Abortive Therapies**

Generic Name	Level of Risk in Pregnancy	Breastfeeding—Hale Lactation Rating
Acetaminophen	B	L1
NSAIDS:Ibuprofen Naproxen	B (D in 3rd trimester)	L1–L2
Metoclopramide	B	L2
Prochlorperazine	C	L3
Magnesium	A (D when used over 5–7 days)	L1
Triptans	C	L3
Dihydroergotamine	X	L4
Codeine	C (D at term)	L3
Butalbital	C	L3
Morphine	B (D at term)	L3
Prednisone	C (D in the 3rd trimester)	L3

TABLE 13.2 **Preventative Medications**

Drug Class	Generic Name	Level of Risk in Pregnancy	Hale Lactation Rating
Beta-blockers	Atenolol	D	L3
	Metoprolol	C (D at term or prolonged use)	L3
	Nadolol	C (D at term or prolonged use)	L4
	Propranolol	C (D at term or prolonged use)	L2
	Timolol	C (D at term or prolonged use)	L2

BOX 13.1 **Emergency Treatment of Migraine in Pregnancy**

A sequential algorithm for migraine treatment:

- Intravenous fluids suggest normal saline at 20–30 mg/kg over 1–2 hours and 500 mg- 1 gm of intravenous, IV magnesium sulfate
- Metoclopramide 10 mg IV or prochlorperazine 5–10 mg IV
- Methylprednisolone 1 gm IV or 6 mg subcutaneous sumatriptan
- Analgesics

KEY POINTS TO REMEMBER

1. Migraines, especially migraine without aura, often go into remission in the second trimester.
2. Migraineurs have an increased risk of eclampsia.
3. Migraines during pregnancy are usually treated with abortive therapy only.
4. Alternative therapies such as biofeedback, stress management, and massage can be helpful adjunctive treatments for certain patients.

References

1. Sances G, Granella F, Nappi Re, et al. Course of migraine during pregnancy and postpartum: a prospective study. *Cephalalgia.* 2003;23:197–205.
2. MacGregor EA. Headache in pregnancy. *Continuum Neurol.* 2014;1(2):128–147.
3. Marcoux S, Bérubé S, Brisson J, et al. History of Migraine and Risk of Pregnancy-Induced Hypertension. Epidemiology 1992;3:53-56.
4. Nezalova-Henriksen K, Spigset O, Nordeng H. Triptan exposure during pregnancy and the risk of major congenital malformations and adverse pregnancy outcomes: results from the Norwegian Mother and Child Cohort Study. *Headache.* 2010;50(4):563–575.
5. Klein AM, Loder E. Postpartum headache. *In J Obstet Anesth.* 2010;19:422–430.

14 A Lady with a Headache in the Second Trimester

M. Angela O'Neal

A 22-year-old lady who is 26 weeks pregnant comes in for evaluation of new headaches over the last several weeks. She has gained 47 lbs. She is currently having headaches primarily in the morning. The headaches are worse with cough or valsalva. She has occasional episodes of blurred vision. On examination, she is 64 inches tall and weighs 230 lbs. Her neurological exam is notable for papilledema.

What do you do now?

IDIOPATHIC INTRACRANIAL HYPERTENSION

Diagnosis

The first concern is to establish the diagnosis. The patient is presenting with symptoms of elevated intracranial pressure (ICP). The differential includes a mass lesion causing elevated ICP, cerebral venous thrombosis (CVT), and idiopathic intracranial hypertension (IIH). The history of significant weight gain and the timing of her symptoms, occurring during the late second and early third trimester of pregnancy, favor IIH.[1] The hypercoagulable state of pregnancy is maximal near the time of delivery and the first six weeks postpartum, so CVT is less likely. The evaluation should include a brain MRI without gadolinium and an MR venogram. The brain MRI is shown is Figure 14.1. The MR venogram was normal. The next step is a lumbar puncture to measure opening pressure. The opening pressure was 300 mm of water. Our patient meets the criteria for diagnosis of IIH.

The International Headache Society 2013 criteria for idiopathic intracranial hypertension are: that the headache should remit after the CSF pressure is in the normal range, CSF pressure is greater than 250 mm, and the majority of patients have papilledema and other symptoms, which may include visual obscurations, pulsatile tinnitus, double vision, and neck or back pain. In addition, other causes of elevated ICP have been excluded.

Complications of Idiopathic Intracranial Hypertension

The major complication of IIH is visual loss. Therefore, the patient needs a neuro- ophthalmology evaluation with visual field testing. She should be followed

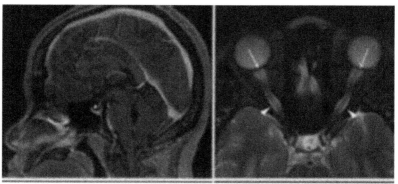

Pictured on the left is a sagittal MRI showing an empty sella. The MRI on the right is an axial flair image showing tortuosity of the optic nerves with dilatation of the perioptic subarachnoid space.

FIGURE 14.1   Brain MRI findings in IIH: Pictured on the left is a sagittal MRI showing an empty sella. The MRI on the right is an axial flair image showing tortuosity of the optic nerves with dilatation of the perioptic subarachnoid space.

by these tests regularly until her ICP is normalized. The risks for visual loss in pregnant women with IIH is the same as in the non-pregnant state.[2]

Treatment

IIH treatment includes weight control, high-volume lumbar punctures, and medications. In pregnancy, moderate weight-reduction is recommended, as ketosis can have adverse fetal consequences. A nutrition consultation was placed to educate the patient and give recommendations about appropriate weight gain.[3]

A high-volume lumbar puncture, removal of 30 cc of cerebrospinal fluid, was performed, as this is a quite effective temporizing measure to normalize the ICP. This can be repeated as needed for symptom control, especially given that she is in the last trimester and her symptoms are likely to improve with the anticipated postpartum weight loss.

In general, the usual medications used to treat IIH are not recommended in pregnancy, as there are limited data to show safety. These medications include acetazolamide, diuretics, and topiramate. A small trial with acetazolamide in the second trimester was reassuring, as the offspring did not have any major congenital malformations. However, the sample size was too small to establish safety.[4] Simple analgesics such as butalbital, acetaminophen and caffeine can be used in limited amounts to help give the patient headache relief.

Obstetrical and Anesthesia Concerns

Excessive weight gain during pregnancy will exacerbate and in some instances trigger IIH, as illustrated in this case. Other pregnancy complications are related to obesity itself, which increases the risk of gestational hypertension, preeclampsia, and gestational diabetes. IIH itself does not cause any fetal complications. The mode of delivery is dictated by the obstetrical issues. There is no contraindication to neuroaxial anesthesia; both spinal and epidural anesthesia are safe and effective.[5] The exception would be when a lumbar shunt is in place for management of the IIH. In that case, there is theoretical concern that neuroaxial anesthesia might damage the shunt.

KEY POINTS TO REMEMBER

1. To establish the diagnosis of IIH requires that other secondary causes of elevated intracranial pressure be excluded such as mass lesions and cerebral venous thrombosis and there must be intracranial hypertension with an opening pressure >250 mm of water.

2. The major complication of IIH is visual loss, so a neuro-ophthalmology evaluation is important.
3. Management of IIH during pregnancy involves weight control and high-volume lumbar punctures rather than medication.
4. The mode of delivery should be dictated by obstretrical concerns.

References

1. Digre KB, Varner MW, Corbett JJ. Pseudotumor cerebri and pregnancy. *Neurology*. 1984 Jun;34(6):721–729.
2. Kesler A, Kuperminc M. Idiopathic intracranial hypertension and pregnancy. *Clin Obstet Gynecol*. 2013;56(2):389–396.
3. Tang RA. Management of idiopathic intracranial hypertension in pregnancy. *MedGenMed*. 2005;7(4):40.
4. Falardeau J, Lobb BM, Golden S, Maxfield SD, et al. The use of acetazolamide during pregnancy in intracranial hypertension patients. *J Neuroophthalmol*. 2013 Mar;33(1):9–12.
5. Bagga R, Jain V, Gupta JR, et al. Choice of Therapy and Mode of Delivery in Idiopathic Intracranial Hypertension During Pregnancy. *MedGenMed*. 2005;7(4):42.

15 Ringing in the Ears and Pain in the Head

M. Angela O'Neal

A 26-year-old lady is referred to you for evaluation of headache. The headache began two days after a vaginal delivery with epidural anesthesia, which required multiple attempts. She has a holocephalic headache, which is worse with sitting or standing and relieved with lying down. She also notes tinnitus, which is worse when sitting up. Her neurological exam is normal.

What do you do now?

LOW-PRESSURE HEADACHE

Pathophysiology

Low cerebrospinal fluid (CSF) volume is felt to cause sagging and traction on the nerves, particularly at the base of the brain. This sagging, when severe, can cause rupture of the bridging veins, leading to a subdural hematoma. Furthermore, sagging of the pons against the clivis may result in cranial nerve palsies. When there is loss of CSF, venous dilation occurs in order to maintain a constant intracranial volume. This pathophysiology explains the MRI findings in low-pressure headache, which include: meningeal enhancement due to venous dilatation, brain sagging that may cause either a tonsillar herniation syndrome or a pseudo-Chiari malformation, which disappears following treatment. The sagging of the brain may also cause apparent pituitary enlargement, and a subdural hematoma can result from the stretching of the bridging veins.

Clinical Characteristics

The classic syndrome is a headache that gets worse in the upright position and disappears after a few minutes of being supine. The most common cause is a postdural puncture headache (PDPH), as in our case. The headache is generally worse at the end of the day, and is often, due to the continuity of the perilymph with CSF, associated with postural tinnitus. However, over time, the patient may not continue to have postural exacerbations. In addition, spontaneous low-pressure headache can occur where there may be no clear triggering event.

Evaluation

In a classic case such as the one presented, no further evaluation is needed. When the diagnosis is unclear, a brain MRI with gadolinium can be helpful in establishing the diagnosis. A lumbar puncture (LP) to check the opening pressure, while it may be necessary is problematic, as it is likely to worsen the headache syndrome.

Risk Factors

Low-pressure headache is much more common in younger individuals and rare after the age of 60. In the 20–30 age group, the incidence of low-pressure headaches has been reported in up to 16% of individuals following a lumbar puncture. This is twice the reported incidence of individuals in the 30–40 age range. PDPH is more common in women. Other risk factors include: a low BMI, a history of migraine, and a prior history of low-pressure headache. The risk of PDPH has been shown to be minimized both by operator experience in minimizing trauma, appropriate orientation of the needle bevel, and by using a smaller-gauge, non-cutting LP needle.[1]

Treatment

The initial recommended treatment is bed rest with good hydration. Many patients' headaches will spontaneously improve with this alone. There has been shown some benefit from using caffeine in treating low-pressure headache. In a randomized controlled trial, 41 patients with refractory PDPH were given IV normal saline versus IV caffeine 500 mg. At two hours, the headache relief was 75% of the caffeine-treated group versus 15% in the normal saline group.[2] The use of oral caffeine 300 mg had marginal benefit in a placebo-controlled trial.[3] Multiple other agents have been tried that show modest benefit, including gabapentin, steroids, and theophylline.[4] Taking the patient's own blood and then injecting it into the epidural space, a "blood patch," is the gold standard of treatment. Ninety percent of patients will have their headache alleviated after a single blood patch, and 96% after a second blood patch.[5]

Our patient was recommended to stay on bed rest for 24 hours and use butalbital, acetaminophen and caffeine 1 tab every four hours. If her headache persisted the following day, she would be offered a blood patch.

KEY POINTS TO REMEMBER

· Low-pressure headaches classically are alleviated after 5 minutes in the supine position.
· The findings on brain MRI reflect the pathophysiology and are related to brain sagging and the compensatory expansion of the venous system.
· A blood patch is the most efficacious treatment.

References

1. Goadsby PJ, Boes C, Sudlow CL. Low CSF volume. *Practical Neurol.* 2002;2:192–197.
2. Jarvis AP, Greenawalt JW, Fagraeus L. Intravenous caffeine for postdural puncture headache. *Anesth Analg.* 1986;65:316–317.
3. Camann WR, Murray RS, Mushlin PS, Lambert DH. Effects of oral caffeine on postdural puncture headache. A double-blind, placebo-controlled trial. *Anesth Analg.* 1990 Feb;70(2):181–184.
4. Basurto OX, Martínez GL, Solà I, Bonfill CX. Drug therapy for treating post-dural puncture headache. *Cochrane Database Syst Rev.* 2011 Aug 10;(8):CD007887. doi:10.1002/14651858.CD007887.pub
5. Taivainen T, Pitkänen M, Tuominen M, et al. Efficacy of epidural blood patch for postdural puncture headache. *Acta Anaesthesiol Scand.* 1993 Oct;37(7):702–705.

16 A Pregnant Woman with Aphasia and Right-Sided Weakness

M. Angela O'Neal

A 28-year-old woman, G2 P1 at 30 weeks' gestation, was last seen well at 10 am. Fifty minutes later, she was found on the ground, not speaking or moving her right side. On examination, her blood pressure was 130/80. She was mute with a left gaze deviation and a dense right hemiplegia. Her non-contrast head CT was normal.

What do you do now?

ISCHEMIC STROKE

Incidence and Etiology of Stroke

Stroke in pregnancy is rare, but it is a significant cause of disability. There are several normal physiological changes that occur in pregnancy that can predispose to stroke. There is a hypercoagulable state associated with pregnancy that occurs in preparation for birth and is maximal near the end of the third trimester and up to six weeks postpartum. This increases the risk of both arterial and venous thrombosis. In women who have a stroke, there is often another underlying hypercoagulable disorder, which when combined with the thrombotic tendency of pregnancy causes a stroke. The hypertension associated with eclampsia is another powerful risk factor for stroke. Eclampsia is associated with both ischemic and hemorrhagic infarcts.

The etiology of stroke during pregnancy is quite diverse. The most common etiology in hospital-based studies is related to cardiac embolism, following which strokes related to eclampsia are the next most common.

Treatment

Tissue plasminogen activator (tPA) is an approved medication for acute stroke in a window of up to four and a half hours following stroke onset.[1,2] In the National

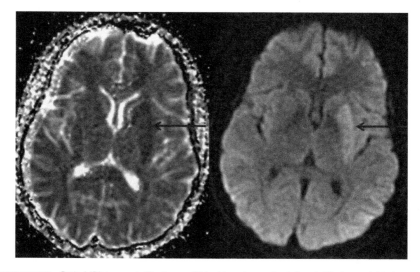

FIGURE 16.1 Brain MRI apparent diffusion coefficient imaging on the left and diffusion-weighted imaging on the right showing an acute infarct in the lenticulostriate territory.

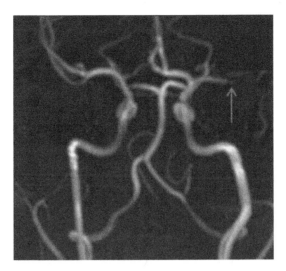

FIGURE 16.2 Brain MRA showing the occlusion of the left middle cerebral artery.

Institute of Health trial, pregnant women were excluded. However, since that time, there have been numerous pregnant women treated with tPA. A review of published studies showed that both maternal and fetal outcomes are generally favorable following treatment with tPA.[3]

The patient received intravenous tPA. She had a brain MRI and neck and brain MR angiogram. The images are shown in Figures 16.1 and 16.2. Her exam did not substantially improve.

What do you do now?
There are now five studies showing efficacy for using intra-arterial (IA) thrombotic retrieval devices in acute stroke.[4-8] There is limited literature for IA therapy in pregnancy using tPA. Again, only case studies and case reports are available. These also support use of IA tPA in pregnancy.[9]

The general recommendation is that the stroke characteristics should dictate the treatment rather than any pregnancy concerns.

KEY POINTS TO REMEMBER

· Stroke in pregnancy is rare, but a substantial cause of morbidity.
· The causes of stroke in pregnancy are diverse.
· Stroke characteristics should guide treatment rather than obstetrical concerns.

References

1. The National Institute of Neurological Disorders and Stroke rt-PA Stroke Study Group. Tissue plasminogen activator for acute ischemic stroke. *N Engl J Med.* 1995;333(24):1581–1587.

2. Hacke W, Markku K, Bluhmki E, et al. Thrombolysis with alteplase 3 to 4.5 hours after acute ischemic stroke. *N Engl J Med.* 2008;359:1317–1329.

3. Dapprich M, Boessenecker W. Fibrinolysis with alteplase in a pregnant woman with stroke. *Cerebrovasc Dis.* 2002;13:290.

4. Berkhemer OA, Fransen PS, Beumer D, et al. A randomized trial of intraarterial treatment for acute ischemic stroke. *N Engl J Med.* 2014;372:11–20.

5. Goyal, M, Demchuk AM, Menon BK, et al. Randomized assessment of rapid endovascular treatment of ischemic stroke. *N Engl J Med.* 2015;372:1019–1030.

6. Campbell BCV, Mitchell PJ, Kleinig TJ, et al. Endovascular therapy for ischemic stroke with perfusion-imaging selection. *N Engl J Med.* 2015;372:1009–1018.

7. Saver JL, Goyal M, Bonafe A, et al. Stent-retriever thrombectomy after intravenous t-PA vs. t-PA alone in stroke. *N Engl J Med.* 2015;372:2285–2295.

8. Jovin TG, Chamorro A, Cobo E, et al. Thrombectomy within 8 hours after symptoms onset in ischemic stroke. *N Engl J Med.* 2015;372:2296–2306.

9. O'Neal MA, Feske SK. Stroke in pregnancy: a case-oriented review. *Pract Neurol.* 2016 Feb;16(1):23–34.

17 Postpartum Visual Disturbance

M. Angela O'Neal

A 35-year-old woman G1 P0 at 31 weeks of gestation woke with a severe headache. She began seeing visual spots, and later completely lost her vision. Shortly thereafter, she developed the worst headache of her life and blacked out. In the emergency department, her blood pressure was 170/120. She received hydralazine 5 mg IV, and labetalol 20 mg IV. Her vision gradually improved. She was transferred to our hospital. Her systolic blood pressure stayed in the 160s. Urinalysis showed 4+proteinuria. She received betamethasone and magnesium. She underwent a caesarean section. A healthy female infant was delivered.

A neurological consult was obtained for intermittent visual symptoms. She reported that the wall seemed to be moving in front of her. Her blood pressure was 160/96. She had a normal neurological exam.

What do you do now?

ECLAMPSIA

Definition

Our patient has the classic symptoms of preeclampsia (PEE). PEE is defined by hypertension, blood pressure greater than 140/90 on two occasions in a previously normotensive woman, and proteinuria—more than 300 mg of protein in a 24-hour urine sample. Eclampsia is defined by seizures and change in mental status. A particularly severe form of PEE occurs when there is liver injury causing hemolytic anemia, elevated liver enzymes and low platelets (HELLP) syndrome. PEE/eclampsia is a major cause of maternal mortality and morbidity. There are also significant fetal consequences, including death, preterm birth, and intrauterine growth restriction.

Pathophysiology

The etiology of PEE is thought to begin by incomplete implantation of the placenta into the uterine myometrium. The abnormal placentation does not allow the spiral arteries in the uterus to develop into a low capacitance system. A milieu of ischemia with a disproportionate ratio of antiangiogenic proteins arises. The result is endothelial injury and hypertension. (1,2) PEE/eclampsia is a multi-organ disorder. The manifestations depend on which end organ is involved. The result of the endothelial dysfunction in the kidney is proteinuria; in the liver, activation of the clotting system resulting in the HELLP syndrome; and in the brain, confusion and seizures. In the brain, the posterior circulation has less ability to autoregulate. In the setting of severe hypertension, the endothelial dysfunction manifests itself by edema, primarily in the parietal and occipital regions. Radiographically, there is white matter edema in the posterior regions of the brain causing the posterior reversible encephalopathy syndrome (PRES). The neurological symptoms of PEE/eclampsia are explained by the part of the brain that is involved. Confusion and visual phenomena are common, related to parietal and occipital lobe injury. Our patient is presenting with symptoms related to PEE/eclampsia. Positive visual symptoms are quite common and should not be attributed to migraine with aura.

Treatment

The presence of the placenta is the driver for PEE/eclampsia. Therefore if a woman is at term when she develops PEE/eclampsia, she should be delivered. The remainder of the treatment is aimed at controlling the blood pressure and preventing seizures. Rapid control of blood pressure is needed, usually with IV

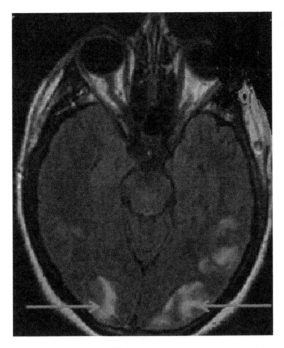

FIGURE 17.1 Brain MRI FLAIR sequence with the arrows depicting posterior white matter changes consistent with posterior reversible encephalopathy syndrome.

labetolol. Several studies have shown that IV magnesium, a 4–6 gram loading dose followed by a maintenance dose of 2 g/hour for 24 hours, is effective in preventing seizures in women with PEE and is more effective than a typical anticonvulsant. (2) The reason that magnesium is more effective may be that beyond its anticonvulsant properties, it acts also as a vasodilator. This patient was treated with IV labetolol and IV magnesium. Brain imaging was recommended (see Figure 17.1).

KEY POINTS TO REMEMBER

1. PEE/eclampsia is a multi-organ disorder caused by endothelial dysfunction.
2. In the brain, the endothelial dysfunction primarily affects the parietal and occipital lobes.
3. The associated radiographic picture is that of PRES.
4. Treatment involves rapid BP control and magnesium to prevent or treat seizures.

References

1. Levin RJ, Lam C, Qian C, et al. Soluble endoglin and other circulating antiangiogenic factors in preeclampsia. *New Engl J Med.* 2006;355:992–1005.
2. Sibai B, Dekker G, Kupferminc M. Pre-eclampsia. *Lancet.* 2015;365:785–799.
3. Lucas MJ, Leveno KJ, Cunningham FG. A comparison of magnesium sulfate with phenytoin for the prevention of eclampsia. *New Engl J Med.* 1995;333:201–205.

18 Postpartum Thunderclap Headache

M. Angela O'Neal

A 39-year-old woman G3 P3 on postpartum day 4 following an urgent caesarian section for hemolytic anemia, elevated liver enzymes, and low platelets (HELLP) syndrome complained of a severe (10/10) bifrontal headache, which was maximal at onset. She was markedly hypertensive with systolic BP in the 230s. Temperature was 37.2°C. Her neurological exam is normal. Imaging is shown in Figure 18.1.

What do you do now?

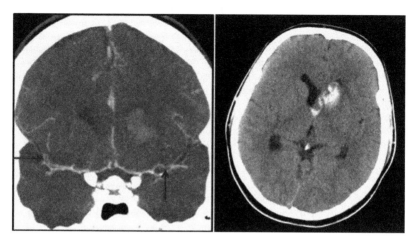

FIGURE 18.1 On the left is the CT angiogram with arrows showing vasoconstriction involving both middle cerebral arteries. On the right is the noncontrast head CT showing a hemorrhage in the left caudate with intraventricular extension.

REVERSIBLE CEREBRAL VASOSPASM SYNDROME

Clinical Features

This lady has reversible cerebral vasospasm syndrome (RCVS). It is manifested by severe "thunderclap" headaches, maximal at onset; and cerebral vasoconstriction, which resolves after 12 weeks. The diagnosis requires seeing vasoconstriction or the so-called string of beads on vascular imaging. Headaches are most common presentation and are typically severe and of a thunderclap nature. They typically last hours and may be recurrent, but generally subside over a month's time. RCVS is a monophasic condition, and most women do well. However, RCVS may cause complications, including seizures; subarachnoid hemorrhage, typically over the hemispheric convexities; and ischemic or hemorrhagic stroke. Due to the vasospasm, ischemic strokes are often located in the watershed or end arterial territories. These complications may cause permanent sequelae.[1]

Pathophysiology

It is felt that RCVS overlaps the posterior reversible encephalopathy syndrome (PRES). Therefore, in pregnancy and postpartum, RCVS is often seen in women who have had eclampsia, like our patient who had a severe manifestation of eclampsia, the HELLP syndrome. The pathophysiology is felt to be related to endothelial dysfunction leading to alterations in vascular tone, causing both expansion and constriction leading to hemorrhage or infarction as well as breakdown of autoregulation, causing PRES.[2]

Precipitants

Many medications have been reported to precipitate RCVS, particularly vaso-active medications such as ergots, amphetamines, cocaine, Lysergic acid diethylamide (LSD), Ecstasy (XTC), immunosuppressants such as tacrolimus, and serotonergic medications-including serotonin reuptake inhibitors, triptans.[3] In the postpartum period, bromocriptine used to stop lactation is a known culprit in vulnerable individuals. Secondary conditions associated with RCVS include the postpartum period, low-pressure headache, carotid endarterectomy, and pheochromocytoma, to name a few.

Treatment

The treatment for RCVS is similar to that of eclampsia: this includes rapid control of blood pressure and intravenous magnesium, even in the absence of eclampsia. In addition, calcium channel blockers seem to help, particularly in symptomatic management of the headaches, although calcium channel blockers do not appear to be effective in modulating vasospasm. Seizures are treated symptomatically. If a precipitating medication is identified, then that should be discontinued and further exposure avoided.

KEY POINTS TO REMEMBER

1. The most common symptom of RCVS is a thunderclap headache.
2. The pathophysiology of RCVS overlaps that which causes PRES, so RCVS is often seen associated with eclampsia.
3. Treatment involves rapid control of blood pressure and IV magnesium. Calcium channel blockers are helpful to manage the headache.

References
1. Ducros A. Reversible cerebral vasoconstriction syndrome. *Lancet Neurol.* 2012 Oct;(10):906–917.
2. Singhal AB. Postpartum angiopathy with reversible posterior leukoencephalopathy. *Arch Neurol.* 2004;61(3):411–416.
3. Ducros A, Bousser MG. Reversible cerebral vasoconstriction syndrome. *Pract Neurol.* 2009 Oct;(5):256–267.

19 Postpartum Left-Sided Numbness and Right-Sided Shaking

M. Angela O'Neal

A 20-year-old woman 10 days postpartum from an uncomplicated caesarian section (C-section) for which she had had epidural anesthesia presents with a diffuse headache. The prior day, she noted left-sided numbness. The day of admission, she had right arm shaking followed by a generalized tonic-clonic seizure. Her BP is 120/90 mm Hg, temperature (T) 97.8°F. She has poor attention consistent with a mild confusional state. There was no focal deficits on examination.

What do you do now?

CEREBRAL VENOUS THROMBOSIS

Clinical Features

The patient by history had a new headache. Subsequently, she had a transient right hemispheric problem causing left-sided numbness. This was followed by a focal seizure with secondary generalization emanating from the left motor cortex. Headache, seizures, and bilateral multifocal localization are the classic findings in a patient with cerebral venous thrombosis. A brain MRI, MR arteriogram, and MR venogram were ordered and confirmed the diagnosis (Figure 19.1). The headaches are related to elevated intracranial pressure and can mimic those of idiopathic intracranial hypertension.

Pathophysiology

Pregnancy is a hypercoagulable state. The changes in coagulation are most prominent in the third trimester and first six weeks postpartum.[1] This is the time when women are at most risk to develop a clotting disorder. These physiological changes occur to minimize bleeding in preparation for birth. Fibrin generation is increased, and fibrinolytic activity is decreased. Levels of factors II, VII, VIII, and X are all increased. Decreases in protein S levels and acquired resistance to activated protein C are common (Figure 19.2). These normal physiological changes contribute to the risk of developing cerebral venous thrombosis (CVT). Other factors associated with an increase in the risk of clotting include infection, fluid loss, inactivity, and C-section.

When CVT occurs, the veins are unable to empty, causing elevated intracranial pressure, seizures, and venous infarcts that are often hemorrhagic. The signs and symptoms of the patient depend on which venous sinus is clotted. Clots in the deep venous system are the most dangerous and have the worst prognosis, as

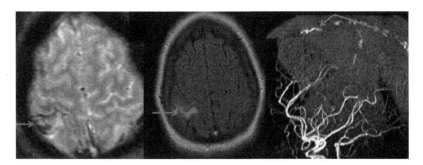

FIGURE 19.1 The image on the left is a gradient ECHO sequence showing susceptibility in the right parietal sulci. The middle image is the FLAIR sequence showing hyperintensity in the same location. These are due to a right parietal vein thrombosis. The image on the right is a brain MRA showing areas of high signal at the superior aspect of the sagittal sinus, consistent with thrombosis.

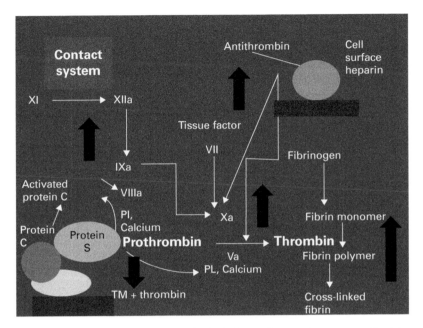

FIGURE 19.2 Depicted are the major changes in clotting factors that occur in pregnancy, ultimately leading to an increase in thrombin production and decreased thrombolytic activity.

these may cause bilateral thalamic lesions. Coma and intracranial hemorrhage are other independent risk factors for a poor prognosis.[2]

Treatment

The treatment for CVT is anticoagulation, even in the presence of hemorrhage. During pregnancy, a heparin derivative is used, as they do not cross the placental barrier. The duration of therapy depends on whether an underlying clotting disorder is found. If no other clotting disorder is discovered, anticoagulation is continued for six months.

Seizures are treated with standard anticonvulsants. It appears that the long-term risk of developing epilepsy is low, especially in the absence of hemorrhage or infarction.

A full hypercoagulable evaluation was done and unremarkable. This patient was started on heparin with a plan to transition to warfarin for six months. She was also loaded with 1 g of levetiracetam.

Future Pregnancies

The risk of complications during future pregnancies is low. On the basis of the evidence, CVT is not a contraindication for future pregnancies. Considering the additional risk that pregnancy confers to women with a history of CVT, prophylaxis with low-molecular-weight heparin during future pregnancies and for six weeks postpartum period is recommended.[3]

KEY POINTS TO REMEMBER

1. Pregnancy is a hypercoagulable state that is most prominent during the last trimester and first six weeks postpartum.
2. Infection, dehydration, inactivity, and having a C-section contribute to an increased risk of clotting
3. CVT is treated with anticoagulation. If no underlying coagulopathy is discovered, full anticoagulation is continued for six months.
4. CVT is not a contraindication to future pregnancies.
5. Women with a history of CVT should be on prophylactic low-molecular heparin during future pregnancies and for six weeks postpartum.

References

1. Kamel H, Babak N, Sriram N, et al. Risk of a thrombotic Event after the 6-Week Postpartum Period. *N Engl J Med.* 2014;370:1307–1315.
2. de Bruijna SF, de Haanb RJ, Stam J. Clinical features and prognostic factors of cerebral venous sinus thrombosis in a prospective series of 59 patients. *J Neurol Neurosurg Psychiatry.* 2001;70:105–108.
3. Saposnik G, Barinagarrementeria F, Brown RD, et al. Diagnosis and management of cerebral venous thrombosis: a statement for healthcare professionals from the American Heart Association/American Stroke Association. *Stroke.* 2011;42:1158–1192.

20 Acute Headache in Pregnancy

M. Angela O'Neal

A 27-year-old female who is currently 29 weeks pregnant is referred for evaluation of an acute headache for nine days. She had previously been worked up for migraines. These headaches have continued to worsen and are refractory to treatment. Her headache continues to be debilitating. Imaging of brain MRI and MR venogram were obtained, which show a pituitary lesion. She woke with a severe 10/10 headache and came to the emergency room (ER) with her husband. A repeat brain MRI was obtained (Figure 20.1).

What do you do now?

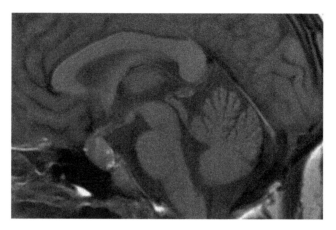

FIGURE 20.1 Sagittal T1 Brain MRI: Expanded pituitary with inhomogeneous intensity within the pituitary. Extension into the suprasellar cistern with compression of optic chiasm.

PITUITARY APOPLEXY

Definition

Pituitary apoplexy is a rare, but potentially life-threatening, condition. It is due to hemorrhagic infarction of the pituitary gland. It is known that this condition is more common with an underlying pituitary adenoma. "Sheehan syndrome" refers to a pituitary necrosis related to blood loss and hypovolemic shock following childbirth.

Anatomy

The pituitary gland sits at the base of the skull in the sella turcica. The anterior pituitary receives blood from the hypothalamus along the infundibulum as venous channels connecting two capillary beds, the so-called portal system. The superior hypophyseal arteries give off branches that supply part of the infundibulum, which receives axons from numerous hypothalamic nuclei. These axons release various releasing and inhibiting factors, which are then taken down the infundibulum via the portal venous plexus and are delivered to the anterior pituitary where they control the release of hormones. The posterior pituitary receives a rich network of arterial supply from the cavernous portion of the internal carotid artery. Due to this unique circulation, pituitary apoplexy can occur in certain circumstances.[1]

The mechanisms postulated include that of a rapidly growing adenoma that outstrips its blood supply. Alternatively, the enlarging mass may compress the portal veins, causing hemorrhagic necrosis. Other risk factors that are associated with pituitary apoplexy include acute changes in blood pressure, stimulation of the gland by increased estrogen states hormonal changes such as pregnancy and coagulopathy. Our patient had a macroadenoma that was rapidly expanding due the hormonal changes associated with pregnancy.[2]

Clinical Features
The most common symptom is headache, which can be severe and thunderclap in nature. It is often referred retro-orbitally due to irritation of the first division of the trigeminal nerve. Other features include involvement of the optic chiasm or optic nerve leading to changes in visual acuity and visual fields. Around 20% of patients will have a change in mental status from a mild encephalopathy to coma. Cranial nerve involvement can commonly occur, related to expansion into the cavernous sinus.

Endocrine Dysfunction
Pituitary apoplexy is a neuroendocrine emergency due hormonal insufficiency. The most important is adrenocorticotropic hormone (ACTH). There are often multiple hormonal deficiencies: growth hormone, hypothyroidism, and hypogonadotropic deficiency. High prolactin levels may reflect a prolactinoma or be due to hypothalamic inhibition. Diabetes insipidus (DI) is also common.

Treatment
The most urgent issue is prompt assessment of fluid and electrolyte imbalance and replacement of corticosteroids. Acute adrenal insufficiency is seen in two-thirds of the patients with pituitary apoplexy and is an important contributor to mortality. The role of surgery versus medical management is controversial.[3] Most would agree that surgery is indicated when there is significant neurological impairment. Our patient was admitted to the neurointensive care unit. She received 100 mg of hydrocortisone immediately and 2.5 mg of bromocriptine. Two days later, she woke with a severe headache, and her visual fields were constricted. After consultation with obstretric-anesthesia and maternal fetal medicine teams, she was taken to the operating room.

Her postoperative course was notable for the fact that she developed DI, complicating her management. She left the hospital to go home nine days after admission. Two months later, she delivered a healthy baby boy.

- Pituitary apoplexy is a neurological emergency.
- The unique vasculature of the pituitary gland makes it vulnerable in certain circumstances to hemorrhage or infarction.
- The neuroendocrine status needs to be assessed immediately.
- Headaches, visual disturbance, and cranial neuropathies involving the nerves in the cavernous sinus are common presenting features.

References

1. Ranabir S, Baruah MP. Pituitary apoplexy. *Indian J Endocrinol Metab*. 2011 Sept;15:188–196.
2. Vargas G, Gonzalez B, Guinto G, et al. Pituitary apoplexy in nonfunctioning pituitary macroadenomas: a case-control study. *Endocr Pract*. 2014 Dec;20(12):1274–1280.
3. Capatina C, Inder W, Karavitaki N, Wass JA. Management of endocrine disease: pituitary tumour apoplexy. *Eur J Endocrinol*. 2015 May;172(5):179–190.

21 The Worst Headache of Her Life

M. Angela O'Neal

A 34-year-old woman G3 P2 at 37 weeks of gestation reported the worst headache of her life. En route to the hospital, she became obtunded and developed aphasia with right-sided weakness. On exam, her BP was 160/90 mm Hg. She could be roused only with a sternal rub. Her speech was nonsensical, and she had a dense right hemiparesis. The platelet count was 250 K, the international normalized ratio, INR 0.9. She had no proteinuria. In the emergency room, she had two generalizing tonic-clonic seizures. She was intubated and transferred to our institution. On arrival, her temperature was 37.1°C, BP 130/85 mm Hg, heart rate (HR) 80. She was unresponsive to sternal rub. She had anisocoria: the left pupil was 4 mm and the right 3 mm. They were reactive to light. Oculocephalic and corneal responses were present. She had decerebrate posturing. Her imaging is shown in Figure 21.1.

What do you do now?

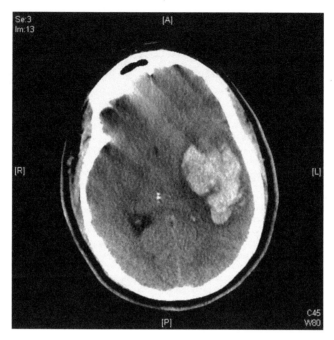

FIGURE 21.1 Plain head CT showing a large frontal temporal bleed.

AVM: ARTERIOVENOUS MALFORMATION

Natural History

The timing of rupture of an arteriovenous malformation, AVM, corresponds to the timing of maximal volume changes during pregnancy. The changes in intravascular volume and cardiac output peak at 25–30 weeks, followed by further increases in cardiac output with labor and delivery and the immediate postpartum period.

Data about if pregnancy confers an increased risk of an AVM rupturing are inconclusive.[1,2] However once there has been a hemorrhage related to an AVM, the risk of re-rupture is high.[3] Therefore, treatment is dictated by best neurosurgical considerations rather than obstetric concerns. Our patient underwent an emergency caesarian and hemicraniectomy, done in tandem. The following day, an arteriogram showed a small AVM with an intranidal aneurysm. She underwent clot evacuation and definitive resection of the AVM (Figure 21.2).

It is recommended that women with known unruptured AVMs be treated prior to becoming pregnant. Stereotactic radiosurgery treatment for an AVM is not recommended in pregnancy, both as it exposes the fetus to radiation and because there is a lag of up to several years prior to seeing a treatment effect on the AVM.[4]

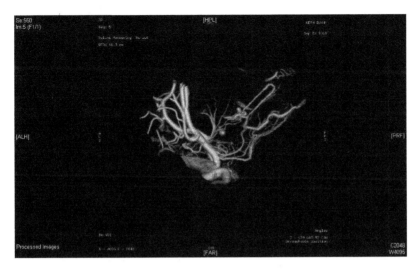

FIGURE 21.2 The arteriogram shows the vascular malformation with a nidal aneurysm.

KEY POINTS TO REMEMBER

1. The timing of rupture of an AVM corresponds to the timing of maximal volume changes in pregnancy.
2. Treatment of a ruptured AVM is based on best neurosurgical practice.
3. An unruptured AVM should be treated prior to pregnancy.

References

1. Gross BA, Du R. Hemorrhage from arteriovenous malformations during pregnancy. *Neurosurgery.* 2012;71:349–355.
2. Horton MC, Chambers WA, Lyons SL, et al. Pregnancy and the risk of hemorrhage from cerebral arteriovenous malformations. *Neurosurgery.* 1990;27:867–871.
3. Liu X, Wang S, Zhao Y, et al. Risk of cerebral arteriovenous malformation rupture during pregnancy and puerperium. *Neurology.* 2014;82:1798–1803.
4. Ogilvy CS, Steig PE, Awad I, et al. Recommendations for the management of intracranial arteriovenous malformations: a statement for health care professionals from a special writing group of the Stroke Council, American Stroke Association. *Stroke.* 2001;32(6):1458–1471.

22 A Woman in Labor with Hypotension and Dyspnea After Epidural Placement

Janet Waters

A 32-year-old female with history of significant obesity presented at 40 weeks' gestation in labor. Blood pressure was 130/80, and pulse was 85. Epidural anesthesia was planned prior to vaginal delivery. Placement was challenging. A test dose of 3 mL of 1.5% lidocaine + epinephrine was given, immediately followed by 10 ml of 0.25% Bupivacaine. About three minutes later, the patient complained of inability to feel or move her legs. She then developed shortness of breath followed by marked hypotension, with systolic blood pressure of 60 and heart rate of 40.

What do I do now?

EPIDURAL AND SPINAL ANESTHESIA

Total spinal block is a rare but serious complication of epidural anesthesia. It occurs when large doses of local anesthetic intended for the epidural space are inadvertently injected into the subarachnoid space. This can produce anesthesia involving the entire spinal cord, nerve roots, and brainstem. When this occurs, patients develop weakness of the lower and sometimes upper extremities. Cranial nerve findings, including pupillary dilatation, may occur. Respiratory insufficiency ensues, followed by cardiovascular collapse with profound hypotension and bradycardia. Instant recognition and supportive treatment is needed to prevent maternal and fetal demise. Patients may be placed in reverse Trendelenburg to prevent further caudal spread of the anesthetic agent. Intubation and positive pressure ventilation can be done to manage respiratory insufficiency. Hypotension may be managed with vasopressors such as epinephrine, norepinephrine, ephedrine, or phenylephrine. Bradycardia can be treated with atropine or glycopyrrolate. Urgent delivery by elective caesarean section may be indicated if fetal bradycardia ensues.

The primary factor that leads to a total spinal block is the failure to wait an adequate time following a test dose. A test dose is a small amount of local anesthetic with epinephrine. This test dose is intended to assess whether an epidural catheter has inadvertently been placed either in a vein or into the intrathecal space. If it has been placed into a vein, then the patient will experience tachycardia from the epinephrine and light-headedness from local anesthetic neurotoxicity. If the catheter is placed into the intrathecal space, the patient will develop lower-extremity paralysis; however, because of the small dose, the block doesn't spread beyond the umbilicus. Following a test dose, three to five minutes should pass prior to larger doses of local anesthetic. If this time is not given, then a total spinal block can result upon further dosing. Given full and immediate support, most patients with a total spinal block have complete recovery with no further sequelae.

Other Complications of Epidural and Spinal Anesthesia

Epidural Hematoma

Epidural hematoma occurs in one out of 200,000 spinal anesthetics and one in 150,000 epidurals. Predisposing risk factors include spinal cord and nerve root tumors, coagulopathy, and inherited and iatrogenic clotting dysfunction. Women with significantly decreased platelet counts due to HELLP are at risk for this complication. Use of antiplatelet agents or anticoagulants can also sharply increase the risk of developing an epidural hematoma. Neuraxial anesthesia must be delayed until the effects of these drugs have subsided (Table 22.1).

TABLE 22.1 Anticoagulants and Waiting Period Prior to Neuraxial Procedure

Medication	Prior to Neuroaxial Procedure
Fondipaparinux (Arixtra)	72 hours
Clopidogrel (Plavix)	48 h
Abciximab (Reopro)	48 h
Enoxaparin (Lovenox) high dose	24 h
Enoxaparin (Lovenox) low dose	12 h
Eptifibatide (Integrelin)	8 h
Tirofiban (Aggrastat)	8 h
Unfractionated heparin, high dose IV continuous	When PTT < 40s
Unfractionated heparin, low dose	No time restrictions

Signs and symptoms of epidural hematoma include unusual back pain, numbness or weakness in the legs, and bowel and bladder dysfunction. Urgent MRI may be used to confirm the diagnosis. Emergency surgical decompression should be undertaken as soon as possible to reduce the risk of permanent injury. Diagnosis can be confounded by prolonged labor where a normal neurological exam is obscured by the presence of epidural anesthesia.

Spinal Cord Injury

Direct spinal cord injury can occur when neuraxial anesthesia is injected into the spinal cord instead of the epidural or subarachnoid space—in 80% of patients, the spinal cord and conus medullaris end at the level of the first lumbar vertebra, and in 20% of patients at the level of the second lumbar vertebra. Placement of the neuraxial block below the L2 level reduces the risk of injury. When this does not occur, direct injury to the spinal cord, conus medullaris, or nerve roots may occur. Patients will complain of pain or paresthesias in the lower extremities when a needle or catheter hits the spinal cord or conus.

Epidural Abscess

Epidural abscess is uncommon and occurs in 1:500,000 neuraxial blocks in the obstetrical population. Onset of symptoms may occur several days after the procedure. Skin flora are the most common infectious agents, with *Staphylococcus aureus* being the most common bacteria. Failure to adhere to aseptic conditions while placing a neuraxial block can increase risk of development. Prolonged use of epidural catheters beyond three days can also raise the incidence of epidural abscess. Immunocompromised patients are also at risk. Patients will present with fever, headache, back pain, leg weakness, and bowel and bladder dysfunction. Urgent MRI with gadolinium may confirm the diagnosis. Aggressive treatment with antibiotics is necessary. In cases of cord compression, surgical decompression may be necessary.

Meningitis

Meningeal infection is a rare complication of epidural and spinal anesthesia. It occurs in 1:39,000 cases. Microbial contamination from the mouth or the nose of the individual performing the block is the most frequent source. *Streptococcus viridans* is the most common agent. Use of face masks and sterile gloves reduces the risk of transmitting infectious agents. Clinical manifestations include headache, fever, neck pain and stiffness, and confusion. Seizures may also occur. Diagnosis is made by lumbar puncture, and treatment is with appropriate antimicrobial therapy.

Intravascular Injection of Local Anesthetic

This complication can occur during epidural anesthesia placement when a large amount of local agent is inadvertently injected into the vascular system. Toxicity to cardiovascular and nervous system ensues. Bupivacaine is the most toxic, followed by ropivacaine, levobupivacaine, lidocaine, and chloroprocaine. Patients may complain of a metallic taste in the mouth, perioral paresthesias, double vision, and tinnitus. Agitation and confusion may occur, followed in some patients by seizures. Cardiac collapse may occur, with hypotension, arrhythmia, and cardiac arrest. Lipid emulsion is the treatment of choice. A 20% intralipid should be given as a 1.5 mL/kg IV bolus over 60 seconds, followed by a 0.25 mL/kg IV (400 ml) infusion over 30–40 minutes. The infusion of lipid may be continued until cardiovascular status stabilizes. Continuation of cardiopulmonary resuscitation is necessary during lipid infusion. Some advocate the use cardiopulmonary bypass if available. Recovery may take up to two hours. As discussed above, the use of a test dose is mandatory in order to avoid this complication.

Dural Puncture Headache

Dural puncture headache is the most common complication of obstetrical anesthesia. It can occur after spinal anesthesia, which is typically used for elective caesarean section. It most commonly occurs when epidural anesthesia is administered for labor pain management and the dura is inadvertently punctured. The larger needle that is used for epidural placement allows greater CSF leakage a smaller spinal needle does. Dural puncture headache results from this CSF leak through the punctured dura. This results in a low-pressure headache. Onset is usually within 24–48 hours of the procedure but can occur up to five days after delivery. Patients experience a diffuse headache upon standing, which improves within 15 minutes after lying flat. Traction on the meninges and meningeal vessels upon standing is felt to be the source of the postural symptoms. Some patients complain of neck stiffness, or tinnitus with an echoing effect. Severe cases may result in 6th nerve palsies with diplopia.

Treatment may be initiated with bed rest and hydration. If the symptoms do not improve after 24–48 hours of conservative management, then an epidural blood patch may be done by the anesthesiology team. This is performed by placing 15–20 ml of autologous blood into the epidural space. The blood serves as a "patch" over the dural hole. The volume of blood may restore central nervous system (CNS) pressure. Patients often experience immediate relief. Success rate is 70–97%. In some patients, a second patch is needed. In patients whose headaches are not postural, other possible diagnoses must be considered and appropriate workup initiated.

KEY POINTS TO REMEMBER

- Total spinal block may be prevented by assuring three to five minutes have passed after giving the test dose of local anesthetic and epinephrine prior to administering full dose of the anesthetic agent.
- Administering neuraxial block below the L2 lumbar level reduces the risk of spinal cord and cauda equina injury.
- Postdural headache is the most common neurological complication of neuraxial block. The hallmark is a headache that improves when the patient is supine. Persisting symptoms may be treated with an epidural blood patch.

References
1. Klein, A. *Neurological Illness in Pregnancy*. Sussex, UK: Wiley Blackwell. 2016:70–79, 153–166.
2. Berger CW, Crosby ET, Grodecki W. North American survey of the management of dural puncture occurring during labour epidural analgesia. *Can J Anaesth*. 1998;45:110–114.
3. Turnbull DK. Shepherd DB. Post dural puncture headache: pathogenesis, prevention and treatment. *Brit J anaesth*. 2003;91:718–729.

4. Crawford JS. Experiences with epidural blood patch. *Anaesthesia*. 1980;35:513–515.
5. Brooks H, May A. Neurologic complications following regional anesthesia in obstetrics. *Brit J anaesth CEPD Rev.* 2003;3:111–114.
6. Scott DB, Hibbard BM. Serious non-fatal complications associated with extradural block in obstetric practice. *Br J Anaesth*. 1990;64:537–541.
7. Dillane D. Finucane B T. Local anesthetic systemic toxicity. *Can J Anaesth*. 2010;57:368–380.
8. Brull SJ. Lipid emulsion for the treatment of local anesthetic toxicity: patient safety implications. *Anesth Analg*. 2008;106:1337–1339.

23 Weakness in the Hand of a Woman During Pregnancy

Janet Waters

The patient is a 37-year-old female at 36 weeks' gestation who presents with complaint of a painful "pins and needles" sensation in her right hand. She reports pain in her forearm as well. It awakens her at night. She obtains some relief by shaking the hand or changing position. Over the past week, she has noted clumsiness of her thumb and difficulty texting on her cell phone. Examination reveals a pregnant female who is normotensive. General exam is notable for pitting edema. She has decreased pinprick in the thumb, index, and third fingers and weakness in abduction and flexion of the thumb of the right hand.

What do I do now?

CARPAL TUNNEL

Carpal tunnel syndrome is a common neuropathy, with an incidence of 3.4% in the general population in the United States. It occurs more frequently in pregnant women than in the general population, with an incidence of Electromyography confirmed cases of 17%. It is the most common mononeuropathy in pregnant women.

Carpal tunnel syndrome is caused by compression of the median nerve as it passes together with the tendons of the hand under the flexor retinaculum. It was first described by Marie and Foix in Paris in 1913. An autopsy performed on a patient with atrophy of thenar muscles revealed neuromas in the median nerve at the level of the transverse carpal ligament. These authors were the first to suggest that a cure for the condition might be achieved by section of the ligament. The surgical procedure did not take place, however, until 1941, when a successful decompression was performed at the Mayo Clinic.

The median nerve has roots in the C5, C6, C7, C8, and T1 vertebrae. In the axilla, the lateral and medial cords of the brachial plexus join to form the median nerve. It enters the cubital fossa and passes between the two heads of the pronator teres. It gives off a branch, the anterior interosseus nerve, which supplies the flexor pollicus longus, the pronator quadratus, and the lateral half of the flexor digitorum profundus. It courses through the distal forearm, and the palmar cutaneous branch emerges as the median nerve becomes superficial above the wrist and supplies sensation to the thenar eminence and central palm. The median nerve continues on and passes through the carpal tunnel and into the hand where it supplies sensation to the palmar surface of the thumb, the first three digits, and the lateral surface of the fourth digit. It also innervates several muscles, including lumbricals I and II, opponens pollicus, abductor pollicus brevis, and flexor pollicus brevis–superficial head. The sides and inferior surfaces of the tunnel are formed by the carpal bones and pronator quadratus. The flexor retinaculum forms the roof of the tunnel. An increase in the volume of the tunnel contents or a decrease in the size of the tunnel may lead to compression of the median nerve at this location.

Patients with carpal tunnel syndrome present with complaints of numbness and tingling, which they may have difficulty localizing precisely. Pain in the forearm may also occur. Symptoms may be brought on by repetitive flexion and extension of the wrists. In more severe cases, patients may develop weakness in the muscles of the thumb and thenar atrophy. Wrist flexion, flexion of the second and third digits, and sensation of the thenar eminence are spared, as the innervation to these areas is provided by nerves that branch off proximal to the carpal tunnel (Box 23.1).

Examination will reveal loss of pinprick sensation in the first three digits and weakness of the abductor pollicus brevis (Figure 23.1). This muscle is best tested by having the patient abduct the thumb perpendicular to the plane of the palm. In the past, neurologists advocated testing for Tinel's sign (tapping over the median nerve as it passes through the carpal tunnel at the wrist) and Phalen's maneuver (allow wrists to fall freely into maximum flexion for 60 seconds) to confirm the diagnosis. The use of these exam techniques has become controversial as studies

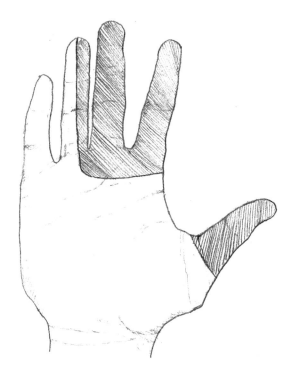

FIGURE 23.1   Sensory loss in carpal tunnel syndrome.
Illustration by J. Risien Waters

have shown that patients with electrodiagnostically evident carpal tunnel syndrome as well as controls may or may not have positive Phalen's and Tinel's signs.

A number of conditions have been associated with increased risk of carpal tunnel syndrome, including Colles fracture, rheumatoid arthritis, diabetes mellitus, hypothyroidism, obesity, and pregnancy. Incidence in diabetics with neuropathy is as high as 30%. Diabetics without neuropathy carry a risk of 14%. Although pregnancy confers higher risk than the general population at 17%, gestational diabetes does not confer additional risk.

Carpal tunnel syndrome in pregnancy presents most often in the third trimester. Nulliparity and edema increase the likelihood of developing the disorder. Gestational fluid retention and increased pressure within the carpal tunnel probably lead to the median nerve compression. Onset in pregnancy is more likely to be bilateral. The diagnosis may be confirmed with electromyography and nerve conduction velocity studies and may be safely done in pregnant women; however, clinical features alone may provide the diagnosis. Conservative management with wrist splints worn at night is effective in over 80% of patients. Local steroid injections can provide relief in patients with severe symptoms that do not respond to splints. Most patients have improvement after delivery. Studies have shown that half of patients have resolution within one year, and two-thirds do within three years.

KEY POINTS TO REMEMBER

- Carpal tunnel syndrome occurs more commonly in pregnant women than the general population.
- It presents most often in the third trimester of pregnancy.
- Increased frequency is probably due to gestational fluid retention causing increased pressure with the carpal tunnel.
- Half of patients experience resolution of symptoms within one year of delivery and two-thirds within three years.
- Conservative management with wrist splints is recommended.

References

1. Massey EW, Guidon AC. Peripheral neuropathies in pregnancy. *Continuum Neurol.* 2014;20(1):100–114.
2. Klein A. *Neurological Illness in Pregnancy.* Sussex, UK: Wiley Blackwell. 2016:70–79, 153–166.
3. Blumenfeld H. *Neuroanatomy Through Clinical Cases.* Sunderland, MA: Sinauer Associates. 2002:339–365.

24 A Woman with Leg Weakness after Delivery

Janet Waters

The patient is a 32-year-old postpartum female who
delivered her first child via vaginal delivery the day before.
An epidural was placed on the first attempt. Labor required
augmentation with Pitocin. After three hours, forceps were
used to assist delivery of an 8 lb. 12 oz. baby boy. The
next morning, the patient got out of bed for the first time
since delivery. When she attempted to walk, her right leg
buckled, and she was unable to ambulate. She reports no
back pain but does note a prickly sensation on her right
upper thigh. She has had no bowel or bladder symptoms.
Examination revealed an epidural catheter insertion site
that was unremarkable and without firmness or tenderness.
Motor exam revealed diminished power 4/5 at the iliopsoas,
5/5 hamstrings, 3/5 quadriceps, 5/5 tibialis anterior,
gastrocnemius, and extensor halluces longus. Sensory exam
revealed loss of pinprick sensation in the right anteromedial
thigh. Reflex exam was notable for an absent right patellar
reflex. All other reflexes were intact. Toes were down-going.

What do I do now?

FEMORAL NEUROPATHY

The femoral nerve arises from the lumbar plexus where nerve roots L2–L4 are joined. It passes between the iliacus and psoas muscles, then courses under the inguinal ligament. During vaginal delivery, the femoral nerve may be compressed by the fetal head at the level of the inguinal ligament. It may also undergo a stretch injury due to hip abduction and external rotation. A prolonged period of time spent in the lithotomy position can increase the risk of femoral nerve injury. Weakness of hip flexion and knee extension can result.

Femoral nerve injury is the most common cause of postpartum leg weakness. It occurs in 2.8 per 100,000 deliveries. In 25% of patients, injury is bilateral, causing significant impairment of mobility in new mothers. Injury to the femoral nerve produces weakness in the quadriceps femoris and in the iliopsoas muscle if the injury occurs proximal to the inguinal ligament. Sensory loss and anesthesia occur in the distribution of the femoral nerve in the anteromedial thigh (Figure 24.1). Knee jerk will be reduced or absent. Most injuries are demyelinative and improve within days to weeks. Treatment includes knee brace and physical therapy. Patients whose symptoms do not improve within three weeks may undergo electromyography and nerve conduction studies for confirmation and prognostication.

Diagnosis of femoral neuropathy can often be made at the bedside by obtaining a thorough history and clinical exam. The differential diagnosis for leg weakness in the postpartum patient is broad, and it is important to distinguish neuropathies from other, more ominous disorders (Box 24.1).

Epidural hematoma is an extremely rare but serious cause of postpartum leg weakness. It occurs in one in 200,000 patients after spinal anesthesia and one in 150,000 patients who receive epidural anesthesia. Patients will complain of back pain and tenderness, prolonged anesthesia with numbness and weakness, and will have sphincter dysfunction. Risk factors include use of antiplatelet agents and anticoagulants, inherited clotting dysfunction, low platelet count, and the presence of spine and nerve root tumors (Box 24.2). Imaging with MRI confirms the diagnosis, and treatment with urgent surgical decompression is indicated to prevent permanent neurological deficit.

Retroperitoneal hematoma can occur postoperatively following caesarean section in the setting of bleeding diathesis or trauma. Spontaneous rupture of the uterine artery may also produce retroperitoneal hematoma. Patients will complain of pain in the back, hip, groin, and abdomen. Leg weakness is caused by compression of the femoral nerve at the iliopsoas gutter. Diagnosis is made with CT of the abdomen and pelvis.

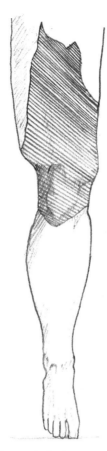

FIGURE 24.1 Sensory loss in femoral nerve distribution.
Illustration by J. Risien Waters

Anterior spinal artery syndrome is an extremely rare entity that can occur in the setting of prolonged hypotension. Lack of perfusion in the anterior spinal artery leads to paraplegia, loss of pain and temperature sensation, and bowel and bladder dysfunction. Proprioception, light touch, and vibratory sense are spared. The presence of bowel and bladder dysfunction and the diffuse weakness and sensory loss distinguish this injury from bilateral neuropathies.

Injury to the conus medullaris during administration of neuraxial block is extremely rare. It occurs if there is inadvertent placement of the catheter at a higher level than L2. Patients will complain of pain in the lower limbs, saddle anesthesia, and bowel and bladder dysfunction. Chemical injury to the cauda equine by local anesthetic agents has been reported and causes lower-extremity weakness, polyradicular pain, numbness, and diminished reflexes. Changes in the anesthetic agents used today have virtually eradicated this complication.

Obstetrical nerve injuries are common and occur in up to 1% of deliveries. The most common lower-extremity nerve injuries associated with pregnancy and delivery involve, in descending order of frequency: the lateral femoral cutaneous nerve, femoral nerve, peroneal nerve, lumbosacral plexus, sciatic nerve, and obturator nerve. Use of epidural anesthesia in the management of labor pain may increase the risk of nerve injury due to its tendency to contribute to prolonged second stage of labor. Absence of sensation prevents women from sensing pressure and adjusting their position. Other risk factors for obstetrical nerve injury include nulliparity, short stature, large fetus, excessive weight gain, and instrumental delivery (Box 24.3).

The most commonly injured nerve in pregnancy is the lateral cutaneous femoral nerve. During pregnancy, it may be stretched or compressed. It is associated with hyperglycemia, excessive weight gain, and large fetal size, and can be a complication of gestational diabetes. Women with this neuropathy complain of painful paresthesias in the lateral thigh. Meralgia paresthetica in pregnancy may be treated by avoidance of tight clothing and positions that aggravate the condition. Most cases resolve after delivery. There is no motor component to the nerve, and it is not a source of postpartum leg weakness.

Injuries to the lumbosacral plexus can occur during delivery due to compression from the fetal head or forceps at the pelvic brim. Symptoms are dependent upon the nerve roots involved. Muscles innervated by L4 and L5 nerve roots are the most affected, causing weakness in ankle dorsiflexion, inversion, and eversion. Sensory impairment is predominantly in the distribution of the L5 dermatome. Achilles reflex is often preserved. Risk factors include large fetal size, small maternal size, fetal malposition, and instrumental delivery.

Fibular neuropathy (previously known as "common peroneal") may be caused by compression of the nerve at the fibular head. In the obstetrical population, it has been attributed to prolonged knee flexion while squatting, lithotomy position, or by pressure on the fibular head during delivery. Patients will develop foot drop due to weakness in the tibialis anterior, extensor hallucis longus, and moderate weakness in foot eversion. Patients will have decreased sensation of pinprick on the dorsum of the foot, most pronounced between the first and second toes. Awareness of the vulnerability to injury has led to appropriate repositioning and decreased frequency of injury.

Obturator neuropathy is rare. It represents less than 4.7% of all postpartum neuropathies. Patients will present with weakness of thigh adduction and sensory loss of the upper third of the medial thigh. Patients with this disorder will have a wide-based gait with circumduction. Risk factors include cephalopelvic disproportion and instrumental vaginal delivery.

Patients are treated supportively with physical therapy.

KEY POINTS TO REMEMBER

- Femoral neuropathy is the most common cause of postpartum leg weakness.
- Hallmarks of femoral neuropathy include legs buckling due to weakness in hip flexors and knee extensors, numbness and paresthesias in the anteromedial thigh, and reduced or absent patellar reflex.

- Postpartum leg weakness due to complication of spinal or epidural placement is exceedingly rare but should be considered in any patient experiencing unusual back pain, radiculopathy, or sphincter dysfunction.

References

1. Massey EW, Guidon AC. Peripheral neuropathies in pregnancy. *Continuum Neurol.* 2014;20(1):100–114.

2. Klein A. *Neurological Illness in Pregnancy.* Sussex, UK: Wiley Blackwell. 2016:70–79, 153–166.

3. Blumenfeld H. *Neuroanatomy Through Clinical Cases.* Sunderland, MA: Sinauer Associates. 2002:339–365.

4. O'Neal A, Chang L, Salajeghi K. Postpartum spinal cord, root, plexus and peripheral nerve injuries involving lower extremities: a practical approach. *Anesth Analg.* 2014;120(1):141–8.

25 A Young Woman with Double Vision and Fatigue

Janet Waters

A 28-year-old female presents with complaints of double vision and fatigue. Examination reveals mild bilateral ptosis, weakness of eye adduction on the left, and proximal muscle weakness in the upper and lower extremities, which worsens with repetitive testing. Serum levels of anti-acetylcholine receptor-binding (AChR) antibodies and anti-muscle-specific kinase (MuSK) antibody titers were normal, but the diagnosis of myasthenia gravis was supported by single-fiber EMG testing and repetitive nerve stimulation studies. Contrast CT of the chest was planned to assess for thymoma. Pregnancy test administered prior to CT was positive.

What do I do now?

MYASTHENIA GRAVIS IN PREGNANCY

Myasthenia gravis is a chronic autoimmune disorder in which antibodies to the postsynaptic neuromuscular junction cause impairment of striated muscle function. It occurs at a case rate of 20 per 100,000 individuals and is more common in women than men, with a ratio of 3:2. It is unmasked or exacerbated in one-third of pregnant women, with worsening symptoms occurring most commonly during the first trimester, the last four weeks of gestation, during delivery, and in the postpartum period. Patients with this disorder experience fluctuating weakness in voluntary muscles leading to ptosis, diplopia, dysphagia, dysarthria, and proximal limb weakness. Diagnosis is confirmed by elevated serum levels of AChR or MuSK antibodies. Seronegative patients may undergo EMG studies with repetitive nerve stimulation and single-fiber studies for confirmation.

There are many issues pertinent to evaluation and treatment of myasthenia gravis in pregnancy. Thymoma is relatively rare in this age group, and even more so in the seronegative population. CT is preferable to MR imaging and may be deferred until after delivery. Thirty percent of patients will undergo exacerbation of their disease during pregnancy, with 20% requiring mechanical ventilation. One-third of pregnant women will experience no change in symptoms and one-third will experience improvement. Having milder symptoms prior to pregnancy does not predict likelihood of worsening or relief from symptoms during gestation.

It is essential to closely follow the patient's respiratory status throughout her pregnancy. The growing fetus may restrict the diaphragm, leading to reduction in lung capacity. Respiratory muscle weakness and fatigue can lead to hypoventilation.

In the first stage of labor, contractions are produced by uterine smooth muscle and are unaffected in women with myasthenia gravis. In the second stage of labor, striated muscle is utilized to expel the fetus. Fatigue can occur, necessitating use of assisted delivery with forceps or vacuum. There is no evidence to suggest that the mode of delivery will affect the likelihood of postpartum exacerbation. The mode of delivery may be based upon obstetrical considerations. Epidural and spinal anesthesia may be used safely in these patients. Regional anesthesia is recommended in patients undergoing caesarean section. If general anesthesia is used, non-depolarizing and curare-like agents should be avoided due to their risk of neuromuscular blockade.

Children born to mothers with myasthenia gravis have no higher risk of developing autoimmune myasthenia gravis. They do have risk of developing transient neonatal myasthenia gravis, which occurs in 4–12% of children born to mothers with myasthenia gravis. In affected children, there is transfer of maternal acetylcholine antibodies across the placenta. Infants may have hypotonia, difficulty with suckling, or respiratory insufficiency. Treatment is supportive with ventilation if indicated. Severe cases may be treated with cholinesterase inhibitors or plasmapheresis. When there is transfer of maternal acetylcholine antibodies in utero, there may be reduction in fetal movements. This can cause polyhydramnios, and in severe cases of infantile paralysis may lead to arthrogryposis multiplex congenita. In this rare disorder, lack of fetal movement causes multiple joint contractures, dysmorphic features, CNS abnormalities, and even stillbirth. Fetal difficulties can occur in a mother with mild symptoms if she produces antibodies to fetal Acetylcholine (Ach) receptors. Mothers who have offspring with fetal complications are more likely to have fetal complications in subsequent pregnancies.

Treatment options in pregnancy must be chosen carefully (Table 25.1). Mild symptoms may require no treatment. Exacerbations may be safely treated with corticosteroids, Intravenous Immunoglobulin (IVIG), or plasmapheresis. Pyridostigmine has been used in pregnancy for symptomatic relief, but there are no controlled studies to confirm its safety. Overuse has been associated with premature labor. Cyclosporine has been associated with increased risk of premature birth, low birth weight, and spontaneous abortion. Infants exposed to Rituximab have been reported to develop B-cell lymphocytopenia. Methotrexate, mycophenalate, and azathioprine have been known to cause a variety of fetal anomalies and loss of pregnancy in the first trimester, and their use should be avoided in patients who are pregnant or who are planning to start a family (Box 25.1).

Patients who have myasthenia gravis have the same risk of developing eclampsia and preeclampsia as does the general population, at 2–8%. While the standard treatment for eclampsia and severe preeclampsia is magnesium, this may not be appropriate for women with myasthenia gravis. Magnesium blocks calcium from entering the nerve terminal and inhibits the release of acetylcholine. This disrupts neuromuscular transmission and may increase muscle weakness. Respiratory distress may follow. Dilantin may be used as an alternative antiepileptic agent in patients with myasthenia gravis.

TABLE 25.1 Therapeutic Interventions in Myasthenia Gravis

Intervention	Side Effects	FDA Pregnancy Category	Teratogenicity
Pyridostigmine	Diarrhea, muscle cramps, cough with increased mucus, bradycardia	C	Probably safe. No controlled studies.
Prednisone	Weight gain, hyperglycemia, hypertension, mood changes, osteoporosis, and myopathy	C	Increased risk of cleft palate in animal studies. Can be used in pregnancy.
Plasma exchange	Hypercoagulability, hypotension, tachycardia, electrolyte imbalances, sepsis, allergic reaction, nausea, vomiting	n/a	Plasma exchange has been used successfully during pregnancy.
Immunoglobulins	Hypercoagulability, headache, aseptic meningitis dermatitis, pulmonary edema, allergic/ anaphylactic reactions	C	IVIG has been used successfully during human pregnancy.
Rituximab	Fever, headache, abdominal pain, hypotension, thrombocytopenia, progressive multifocal encephalopathy	C	B-cell lymphocytopenia generally lasting less than 6 months can occur in infants exposed to rituximab in utero.
Cyclosporine	Renal toxicity, hypertension, seizures, myopathy, increased risk of infections	C	Human studies demonstrate evidence of premature birth and low birth weight for gestational age.

TABLE 25.1 Continued

Intervention	Side Effects	FDA Pregnancy Category	Teratogenicity
Mycophenolate mofetil	Increased risk of infection. Possible increased risk of lymphoma and skin cancer	D	Pregnancy loss in first trimester and congenital malformations in the face and distal limbs, heart, esophagus, and kidney have been reported.
Azathioprine	Hepatoxicity, bone marrow suppression, nausea, vomiting, diarrhea, possible increased risk of lymphoma and leukemia	D	Congenital defects, including cerebral palsy, cardiovascular defects, hypospadias, cerebral hemorrhage, polydactyly, and hypothyroidism.

BOX 25.1 **Medications Known to Exacerbate Symptoms of Myasthenia Gravis**

Marked contraindication:
D-penicillamine and a-interferon cause increased weakness and should not be used in patients with myasthenia gravis.
Relative contraindication. Avoid if possible:

- Succinylcholine, d-tubocurarine, vecuronium, and other neuromuscular blocking agents, including botulinum toxins
- Quinine, quinidine, and procainamide
- Beta-blockers, including propranolol, atenolol, and timelol maleate eye drops
- Calcium channel blockers
- Iodinated contrast agents
- Magnesium, including milk of magnesia, antacids containing magnesium hydroxide, and magnesium sulfate
- Select antibiotics, including:
  - Aminoglycosides (e.g., tobramycin, gentamycin, kanamycin, neomycin, streptomycin)
  - Macrolides (e.g., erythromycin, azithromycin, telithromycin)
  - Colistin

1. In pregnancy, myasthenia gravis symptoms worsens in 30% of women, with 20% requiring ventilator support.
2. Exacerbations occur most often in the first trimester, final four weeks of gestation, delivery, and post-partum period.
3. Corticosteroids, IVIG, and plasma exchange may be used to treat exacerbation in the pregnant population.
4. Azathioprine, mycophenolate mofetil, and methotrexate are contraindicated in pregnancy.
5. The first stage of labor is unaffected by myasthenia gravis, but in the second stage of labor, assisted delivery may be necessary.
6. Regional anesthesia is safe and preferable to general anesthesia.
7. Thymoma is less common in this age group, and imaging with CT may be delayed until after delivery.
8. Use of magnesium in patients with myasthenia gravis may lead to increased muscle weakness and respiratory compromise. Dilantin may be used as an alternative antiepileptic agent.

References
1. Massey JM, De Jesus-Acosta C. Pregnancy and myasthenia gravis. *Continuum Neurol.* 2014;20(1):115–127.
2. Klein A. *Neurological Illness in Pregnancy.* Sussex, UK: Wiley Blackwell. 2016:70–79, 154–158.
3. Bradley G, Daroff R, Fenichel G, Jankovic J. *Neurology in Clinical Practice*, 5th ed. Philadelphia, PA: Butterworth Heinemann Elsevier. 2008:2383–2396.

26 Multiple Sclerosis

Tamara B. Kaplan and Marcelo Matiello

A 31-year-old woman was recently diagnosed with multiple sclerosis (MS) after she suffered from optic neuritis that completely resolved, and had a MRI that fulfilled the 2010 McDonald diagnostic criteria. She would like to hold off on starting any disease modifying therapy (DMT) until after she has a child, as she and her husband are trying to conceive. She becomes pregnant three months later, and her pregnancy is uneventful. She starts breast-feeding, and one month after delivery, she notices tingling and numbness in her lower extremities and has difficulty walking. She is treated with intravenous (IV) methylprednisolone for five days and is able to continue breast-feeding during this period by "pumping and dumping." She stops breast-feeding at six months and is started on glatiramer acetate. Two years later, she desires to get pregnant again.

What do you do now?

MULTIPLE SCLEROSIS IN PREGNANCY

Natural History

A significant number of MS patients will develop the disease during their child-bearing years. Up until the 1950s, women with MS were told that pregnancy could worsen their disease and were discouraged from becoming pregnant; however, based on studies over the past few decades, this information proved to be incorrect.

There was a major shift in thinking with the 1998 publication of the Pregnancy in Multiple Sclerosis (PRIMS) study, which is the best large-scale prospective study published to date. PRIMS included 254 women (246 with relapsing MS), and 269 pregnancies. Patients were followed for at least 12 months postpartum.

Compared to prepregnancy, annualized relapse rate fell by 70% during the third trimester. However, during the first three months postpartum, the relapse rate rebounded to 70% above the prepregnancy level, but then came down and stayed down at the prepregnancy rate after those initial three months. The annualized relapse rate from postpartum months 3–12 was not significantly different from that of the prepregnancy year.

A follow-up study to PRIMS looked at factors that predicted a relapse and found that the risk for postpartum relapse was greatest in those who had experienced a relapse in the year prior to pregnancy or during pregnancy. The findings of the PRIMS study have been replicated by numerous other studies since its initial publication.

How to Treat a Relapse During Pregnancy

When there is concern for worsening disease activity during pregnancy, it is important to rule out factors that may cause "pseudo-exacerbations" such as urinary tract infections, which are more common in pregnancy.

If a relapse is severe enough to warrant therapy, most clinicians will use IV methylprednisolone. This particular corticosteroid is preferred because it is metabolized before crossing the placenta. In general, it is recommended that steroids be avoided during the first trimester, as there are data for increased risk of cleft palate during this period. Other clinicians may use IV immunoglobulin (IVIG), which is safe during pregnancy.

Avoiding Postpartum Relapses

In general, is it advised to resume immunomodulating therapy as soon as possible. For some women, this means after they finish breast-feeding. Other women defer breast-feeding and resume their therapy immediately.

One study showed that monthly steroid infusions for the first six months postpartum seemed to reduce the relapse rate. However, there was no difference in overall neurological function or progression of disease between those treated and controls. Overall, using frequent IV steroids in the postpartum period is not the standard of care, and the use of such therapy should be on an individual basis.

There is minimal transfer of steroids into breast milk. However, regardless, it is recommended that breast-feeding mothers pump and discard their milk, or "pump and dump" and wait for at least four hours after each steroid infusion before resuming breast-feeding.

Use of Disease-Modifying Therapy

Choosing when to stop DMT prior to conception can be a difficult decision for many women with MS. While there may be potential risks in conceiving while on a DMT, there may also be a risk of relapse if therapy is withheld for too long.

According to the U.S. Food and Drug Administration (FDA) and the National MS Society consensus statements, DMTs should not be used in MS patients who are pregnant, trying to become pregnant, or breast-feeding. While there are limited data in humans, some of these medications have been shown to be teratogenic in animal studies (Table 26.1).

There are no specific guidelines regarding the stopping of a DMT before trying to become pregnant. It is thought that one to two months is reasonable for interferon β, glatiramer acetate, and dimethyl fumarate, and two months for fingolimod. Three months have been recommended with natalizumab; however, this is debated as some experts feel that one month's cessation may be sufficient.

Interferons (Rebif®, Avonex®, Bestaseron®, Plegridy®): Interferon βs are the oldest class of DMTs. In primates, there appeared to be a dose-response increase in spontaneous abortions when primates were given doses as high as 40 times the normal dose. This effect has not been seen in humans. There is no animal evidence of teratogenicity, and the large macromolecule is unlikely to be able to cross the placenta in any significant amount.

Glatiramer Acetate (Copaxone®): Glatiramer acetate is the only DMT with the pregnancy "category B." It has been safe in animals, and thus far in over 500 human pregnancies, there has been no association with low birth weight, congenital anomaly, preterm birth, or spontaneous abortion. Currently, some neurologists treat women with glatiramer acetate during pregnancy. Glatiramer acetate does not cross the placenta, and it may also be considered safe with breast-feeding, because it is thought that such a large amino acid polymer is unlikely to be readily absorbed through an infant's gastrointestinal tract.

TABLE 26.1 **Safety of Disease-Modifying Therapies in Pregnancy**

Drug	Pregnancy Category	Teratogenic Risk in Animal Studies	Data in Exposed Humans
Interferons	C	No	No evidence for spontaneous abortion or birth defects
Glatiramer acetate	B	No	No evidence for spontaneous abortion or birth defects
Fingolimod	C	Yes	Some reports of birth defects, but no specific pattern
Dimethyl fumerate	C	No	No evidence for spontaneous abortion or birth defects
Teriflunomide	X	Yes	Needs to be washed out with elimination procedure
Natalizumab	C	No	Possible risk of spontaneous abortion
Alemtuzumab	C	No	Thyroid monitoring necessary for mother throughout pregnancy. No evidence for spontaneous abortion or birth defects
Rituximab	C	No	Risk of B-cell depletion in newborn, thought to be transient

Dimethyl Fumarate (Tecfidera®): Evidence from animal studies suggests that dimethyl fumarate does cross the placenta. Animals, given the highest dose tested, showed an increased rate of spontaneous abortion as well as lower fetal weight and delayed ossification. Despite these studies, in a case series of 45 women exposed to dimethyl fumarate in early pregnancy, there were no significant adverse effects found.

Fingolimod (Gilenya®): Fingolimod crosses the placenta and is secreted in breast milk. In animal studies, there is evidence for both teratogenicity and embryolethality. Fetal malformations and complications included ventricular septal defect, persistent truncus arteriosus, and fetal death. In a limited number of human pregnancies, there seems to be a slightly higher rate of spontaneous abortion, as well as malformations such as acrania, a malformation of the tibia, and tetralogy of Fallot. Currently, it is advised that patients stop fingolimod use at least two months prior to conceiving.

Teriflunomide (Aubagio®): In animal studies, teriflunomide had significant teratogenicity, causing fetal abnormalities such as craniofacial, axial, and appendicular skeletal malformations in pregnant rats and rabbits. Despite these findings, of the recorded human pregnancies with exposure to teriflunomide, the rate of spontaneous abortion was not different from the general population, and no serious malformations were reported. However, caution is still advised. In addition to its ability to cross the placenta, teriflunomide is also present in the semen of men taking the drug. Teriflunomide may stay present in the body for as long as 24 months, but it can be eliminated with a washout protocol using cholestyramine to eliminate the drug.

Natalizumab (Tysabri®): According to the Tysabri Pregnancy Exposure Registry, which reported 375 pregnancies, resulting in 314 live births, the rates of miscarriage and malformation were not increased compared to the general population. However, in animal studies, supratherapeutic doses of natalizumab have been shown to decrease fertility and reduce neonatal survival. Natalizumab crosses the placenta in the second trimester and is secreted at low levels in breast milk. However, it is unclear whether this monoclonal antibody is absorbed through the infant's gastrointestinal mucosa.

Rituximab (Rituxan®): Over the last few years, rituximab has been used more frequently as an off-label treatment for MS, and, if approved, the humanized analogue, ocrelizumab, is likely to be used as well. Rituximab does cross the placenta according to evidence from animal studies; however, these studies showed no evidence of increased risk of miscarriage or teratogenicity. One effect that has been seen in both animal studies and humans is transient newborn B-cell depletion. The risk of B-cell depletion in the newborn appears to be higher when the mother is exposed to the drug during the second or third trimester.

Alemtuzumab (Lemtrada®): This medication is only used in patients with very aggressive or refractory MS. In animal studies, early administration of alemtuxumab resulted in increased rates of fetal loss, as well as decreased B- and T-lymphocytes at birth. It is advised that women should avoid conception for at least four months after the infusion. In a case series of 104 human patients treated with alemtuzumab and 139 pregnancies, there were no increased rates of miscarriage or malformations observed. Almost all of these pregnancies (except six) were conceived at least four months after the alemtuzumab infusion. There was one case of neonatal thyrotoxic crisis that resolved with appropriate treatment. Of note, alemtuzumab is present in the milk of lactating mice treated with this drug.

Breast-feeding

Recently, several studies have suggested that breast-feeding may influence postpartum relapse rate, but the true effect continues to be debated. A small study of women with MS suggested that exclusive breast-feeding might protect against postpartum relapse, possibly through promoting ongoing anti-inflammatory changes. However, a similar study with a much larger pregnancy cohort failed to produce the same findings. Additionally, in the PRIMS study, breast-feeding was ultimately considered to have no effect on postpartum relapses or disability. Some suggest that, while women who breast-feed appear to do better, they may be preselected for those with milder disease. Further research is needed to assess whether breast-feeding may alter postpartum MRI disease activity.

Although there are still many questions, the available evidence suggests that breast-feeding is safe and possibly even beneficial for MS patients. Therefore, while each case should be considered individually, the choice to breast-feed should be generally supported. However, breast-feeding mothers are also advised not to start DMT after birth, as there are limited data available on drug transfer into milk and the effects on newborns.

Assisted Reproductive Technology in MS

In general, MS patients are not thought to have decreased fertility as a result of the disease. However, many MS patients are turning to assisted reproductive technology (ART) for various reasons, including delays in childbearing due to their disease and sexual dysfunction.

To date, no large studies exist of the effect of ART on MS. However, a few small published case series have suggested that there may be an increased risk of relapse with certain forms of ART. In a study of 16 patients who received gonadotropin-releasing hormone (GnRH) agonists and recombinant follicle-stimulating hormone (FSH), it was noted that there was a seven-fold increase in the risk of MS exacerbation, and a nine-fold increase in the risk of enhanced disease activity on MRI. Failure of in vitro fertilization (IVF) has also been shown to be associated with an increased relapse rate. This may be due to a change in hormones that resembles that of the postpartum period. Further research is needed to appropriately advise patients hoping to use ART.

Counseling Women on MS Risk in Their Children

Like many other diseases, MS is thought to occur due to some combination of genes and environmental risk factors. Children of women with MS have a 3–5% lifetime risk of developing the disease. While this is more than the general public with no family history, it also means that there is a 95–97% chance a child will not be affected. Clinicians can provide patients with the facts and statistics, but there is still a lot to be learned, and this is currently an active area of research.

KEY POINTS TO REMEMBER

1. The rate of relapse in MS decreases during pregnancy, especially during the third trimester, but there is a significant increase in relapse rate in the first three months postpartum.
2. Disease-modifying therapies are generally discontinued during preconception, pregnancy, and while breast-feeding.
3. Exclusive breast-feeding may have a beneficial effect in decreasing the postpartum risk of relapse.

References

1. Confavreux C, Hutchinson M, Hours MM, et al. Rate of pregnancy-related relapse in multiple sclerosis. Pregnancy in Multiple Sclerosis Group. *N Engl J Med*. 1998;339(5):285–2291.
2. Vukusic S, Hutchinson M, Hours M, et al. Pregnancy and multiple sclerosis (the PRIMS study): clinical predictors of post-partum relapse. *Brain*. 2004;127(pt 6):1353–1360.
3. Hellwig K, Haghikia A, Rockhoff M, Gold R. Multiple sclerosis and pregnancy: experience from a nationwide database in Germany. *Ther Adv Neurol Disord*. 2012;5(5):247–253.
4. Correale J, Farez MF, Ysrraelit MC. Increase in multiple sclerosis activity after assisted reproduction technology. *Ann Neurol*. 2012;72(5):682–694.

27 A Mother Who Could Not See Her Baby

Marcelo Matiello and Tamara B. Kaplan

A 30-year-old woman, at 28 weeks' gestation of her first pregnancy, was brought to the ED because she was "not feeling well" and was ultimately diagnosed with severe preeclampsia. She subsequently had a caesarian-section. Three weeks postpartum, she had nausea and vomiting, and on her 26th day postpartum, she woke up with decreased vision in her right eye ("80% dark"), with further worsening in the following few days. She was evaluated at the ophthalmology office, and her visual acuity (VA) was finger-counting right eye (OD) and 20/15 left eye (OS). MRI of the brain revealed right optic neuritis (ON). The diagnosis formulation at that time was of lactational ON, and treatment was deferred until her outpatient visit to the neurology clinic. Two weeks after the onset of right ON, she developed new left-eye blurry vision. In the ED, her VA on the OS was 20/200 and only hand waving in OD. She was admitted and treated with IV steroids but had no clinical improvement by day 3. Plasmapheresis was initiated, and by the third session, she obtained significant improvement, with OS 20/30 and OD 20/80. Her laboratory workup was notable for seropositivity for anti-AQP4 antibodies.

What do you do now?

NEUROMYELITIS OPTICA SPECTRUM DISORDERS IN PREGNANCY

AQP4 Antibodies Are the Hallmark of Neuromyelitis Optica Spectrum Disorders (NMOSD)

NMOSD belong to a group of relapsing neurological syndromes characterized by significant morbidity and mortality. The disease happens due to CNS inflammation and necrosis, which is, in most cases, mediated by antibodies (abs) targeting Aquaporin-4 (AQP4).

AQP4 is a water channel present in many tissues (CNS, kidneys, muscle, and others) but most greatly expressed on the foot processes of astrocytes. When compared to other organs, CNS has a much larger content of AQP4, especially in optic nerves, the spinal cord, and certain areas of the brain stem. Along with differences in complement cascade regulation in the CNS compared to other tissues, the greater expression of AQP4 is probably responsible for the disease's common manifestations of optic neuritis, transverse myelitis, and area postrema syndrome (intractable nausea/vomiting and/or hiccups). Other brainstem syndromes, narcolepsy and symptomatic cerebral lesions, are also possible but much less common.

Clinical Clues in NMOSD

NMOSD shows a marked female preponderance (6F:1M) and may affect patients of childbearing age. Compared to multiple sclerosis (MS), NMOSD is also more common in non-white populations. As exemplified by the case of the 30-year-old patient, the consideration of a potential diagnosis of NMOSD begins with an indicative clinical syndrome. It is likely that if she had presented to a neurologist first, she would have been tested for AQP4 antibodies and treated with steroids immediately. NMOSD usually leads to a more severe ON (VA less than 20/200) with poor recovery, and the optic nerve lesions are more likely to be extensive and with chiasmatic involvement compared to optic neuritis in MS.

Patients who are seropositive for anti-AQP4 antibodies (also known as NMO-IgG) are very likely to have NMOSD relapses. The typical myelitis in NMOSD is complete (motor, sensory, and loss of sphincter control) and longitudinally extensive (more than three spinal cord segments). In contrast, MS patients most often have partial spinal cord syndromes, often with sensory abnormalities only. MS-related spinal cord lesions are usually small and peripherally located. Pain and paroxysmal tonic spasms are also more frequent as a result of NMOSD.

The area postrema syndrome happens in almost half of NMO patients along the disease course, often as the initial presentation. "Intractable" nausea, vomiting, and hiccups may occur in isolation or herald the onset of other syndromes, as it happened with our patient.

Planning Pregnancy (I): NMOSD Increases Risk of Miscarriages and Preeclampsia

Pertinent to family planning, presumably NMOSD is due to complex susceptibility; i.e., interaction of multiple genetic and environmental factors, which are largely unknown. Only about 3% of the NMOSD patients also have a relative with the disease.

When counseling a patient with NMOSD who wants to get pregnant, the risk of complications must be discussed. In a study of 40 AQP4-seropositive women with 85 informative pregnancies, there were 11 pregnancies (13%) that ended in miscarriages (Nour et al., 2016). Of those, seven were in the first trimester, one in the second trimester, and three at an unknown time within the first 24 weeks. Six of 14 pregnancies (43%) after NMOSD clinical onset ended in miscarriages, compared to five of 71 pregnancies (7%) that happened before NMOSD onset. In the studied cohort, there was no association between antiphospholipid antibodies and miscarriage rates. It is likely that patients with more "active" disease will have more complications. The mean annualized relapse ratio (ARR) from the nine months preconception to the end of pregnancy was higher in the miscarriage subgroup than in the viable pregnancy subgroup (0.707 vs. 0.100, $p = 0.01$).

Pertinent to the case described, in the same NMOSD pregnancy study, 113 informative pregnancies in 57 women were included in the analysis of the influence of NMOSD on the risk of preeclampsia. The authors found that 13 cases of preeclampsia were distributed among 11 women, corresponding to a preeclampsia rate of 11%. The incidence of preeclampsia in pregnancies occurring before and after NMOSD was similar. Miscarriage in the most recent pregnancy and the presence of multiple other autoimmune diseases were associated with an increased risk of preeclampsia, and no significant association was found between preeclampsia risk and maternal age.

Placenta expresses AQP4, and autoimmunity may be responsible for the pathogenesis of preeclampsia and/or miscarriages. Placental AQP4 expression is high during mid-gestation and progressively decreases with advancing pregnancy. In animal studies, injected anti-AQP4 antibodies bind to mouse placental aquaporin-4, activate proteins of the complement system and cause inflammatory cell infiltration into the placenta, leading to tissue necrosis.

Planning Pregnancy (II): Increased Risk of NMOSD Relapses Postpartum

Besides having an increased the risk of a problematic pregnancy, patients with NMOSD also have higher chances to have relapses in first three months of the postpartum period, compared to zero to nine months preconception. Withdrawal of pregnancy-related immunological tolerance mechanisms mediated by regulatory T cells may induce an immunological and clinical rebound effect and explain such increase of relapses.

NMOSD Management During Pregnancy and Postpartum

There is no FDA-approved treatment for NMOSD due to the lack of completed clinical trials in this disease. However, there are three ongoing trials and other drugs in the development pipeline as of this writing.

Based on case series and expert opinion, treating NMOSD attacks with steroids and plasmapheresis during pregnancy or postpartum is appropriate, and the incidence of side effects or complications of such therapies does not seem to be affected by pregnancy. It is generally recommended to treat an NMOSD attack with five days of 1 g of IV methylprednisolone, and if no significant and immediate response is seen, patients should be started on plasmapheresis sessions every other day for a total of five to seven exchanges.

Immunosuppressive agents are the mainstream method of preventing attacks related to NMOSD. Most medications used to treat NMO have potentially severe toxicities to the fetus. Azathioprine and micophenolate mofetil are classified as pregnancy category D; the usual recommendation is that these medications should not be used without concurrent contraception. Although glucocorticoids and rituximab are pregnancy category C, in general, it is also recommended to discontinue their use in anticipation of pregnancy. However, available data from literature and from registries of other antibody-mediated diseases shows that azathioprine and steroids may be taken by pregnant and lactating women without causing measurable harm to the children. It was also recently reported in two cases of NMOSD that rituximab was compatible with pregnancy and caused only transient immunodeficiency in the child. The use of such medications before and during pregnancy to reduce the risk of disease activity and potentially improve pregnancy outcomes is plausible, but the risk–benefit ratio needs to be discussed in detail with each patient.

If a patient is in good control of her disease (no relapses for at least a year) and decides to become pregnant, she should undergo monitoring for preeclampsia and NMOSD relapses. Immunosuppression should be resumed as soon as delivery occurs, and it is preferable to use rituximab or the combination of azathioprine or micophenolate mofetil with oral steroids.

There are no studies about lactation and NMOSD. The concentration of any IgG in breast milk is very low and generally not absorbed through the intestinal mucosa of the baby. Regarding the common medications used in NMOSD, steroids and azathioprine are detected in breast milk, rarely causing transient neutropenia to the baby. To increase safety, in patients taking more than 50 mg of prednisone, the mother should have a four-hour delay between the prednisone dose and breast-feeding.

KEY POINTS TO REMEMBER

- NMOSD is a severe neurological disease, and pathogenic anti-Aquaporin 4 antibodies are present in most patients.
- NMOSD increases the risk of miscarriages and pre-eclampsia.
- Patients with NMOSD have a higher risk of relapses in the first three months postpartum.
- Immunosuppression is the mainstream method of treatment of NMOSD and should be resumed after delivery.

References

1. Götestam Skorpen C, et al. The EULAR points to consider for use of antirheumatic drugs before pregnancy, and during pregnancy and lactation. *Ann Rheum Dis.* 2016;75:795–810. doi:10.1136/annrheumdis-2015-208840

2. Nour M, et al. Pregnancy outcomes in aquaporin-4–positive neuromyelitis optica spectrum disorder. *Neurology.* 2016 Jan 5;86(1):79–87.

3. Vodopivec I, et al. Treatment of neuromyelitis optica. *Curr Opin Ophthalmol.* 2015 Nov;26(6):476–483. do

4. Matiello M. Aquaporin 4 expression and tissue susceptibility to neuromyelitis optica. *JAMA Neurol.* 2013 Sep 1;70(9):1118–1125. doi:10.1001/jamaneurol.2013.3124

28 "I Am Pregnant; Why Can't I Sleep?"

Sandra L. Horowitz

A 37-year-old woman, seven months pregnant, presents in your office with insomnia. Before this, her third pregnancy, there were no sleep complaints. She has developed snoring in the supine position. For the last month she describes difficulty staying asleep, with daytime sleepiness. She narrowly missed falling asleep at the wheel with children in the car. When she relaxes in the evening, she has sensations in her legs that make it difficult for her to sit still, and this continues in bed, impeding sleep. She describes a feeling of ants crawling on her legs that compels her to get up and walk around the room. It recurs when she returns to bed, but eventually abates around 3:00 am. Wake time is 6:30 am with her other children. She is asking for sleeping pills, as her obstetrician does not want to prescribe them.

Exam is unremarkable, with blood pressure 140/82 mmHg and pulse 64 BPM. BMI is 34. Oral airway is crowded, with a long uvula and prominent posterior tonsillar folds allowing little space in the back of the oropharynx. She has some nasal congestion, and tonsils are not large.

What do you do now?

INSOMNIA

Sleep problems in women are very common, according to a National Sleep Foundation poll,[1] with only 39% reporting good sleep almost every night, and 34% having trouble falling or staying asleep at least a few nights a week. During pregnancy and postpartum, 84% of women report poor sleep at least a few nights a week.

Hormonal changes have an effect on sleep from the first trimester of pregnancy with an 0.7-hour increase in sleep time, related to rises in estrogen and progesterone.[2] Progesterone acts through the GABA receptor, resulting in hypnotic effects in animals, decreasing sleep latency, and increasing non-REM (rapid eye movement) sleep. It also stimulates the respiratory drive and enhances brain sensitivity to carbon dioxide (CO_2). Estrogen suppresses REM sleep by increasing brainstem norepinephrine turnover while it affects nasal mucosa with swelling, leading to obstruction, rhinitis, and snoring. Sleep efficiency decreases early in pregnancy due to nausea, leg cramps, increased urinary frequency, and breast tenderness. By the third trimester, snoring, heartburn, trouble finding a comfortable position, low back pain, fetal movement, nasopharyngeal edema, and restless legs can interfere with sleep. Functional residual capacity (FRC) decreases by 20% from upward pressure on the diaphragm. Snoring is reported in up to 35% of patients during pregnancy with elevation of the apnea hypopnea index, although not to pathological levels in most patients.[3] There is an association of sleep apnea and pregnancy-induced hypertension, with increased adverse outcomes of pregnancy, including fetal growth retardation and premature birth. It has been suggested that treating nocturnal airflow limitation may improve gestational hypertension.[4]

In this patient, her elevated BMI and snoring with daytime sleepiness are signs sleep apnea may be interfering with her sleep (Table 28.1). A polysomnogram or home sleep apnea test would resolve this, and CPAP (continuous positive airway pressure) is useful during pregnancy. Due to the complaint of leg symptoms, an in-lab polysomnogram is preferable, but not always obtainable.

If she had Chronic Insomnia Disorder (ICD-10-CM code: F51.01), the most common complaint is difficulty staying asleep, with early morning awakening next, and problems initiating sleep less frequent.[5] Insomnia treatment in general and especially during pregnancy involves sleep hygiene practices: avoiding caffeine, keeping the bedroom dark and quiet and cool, not exercising too close to bedtime, avoiding media for two hours before bed, and not going to bed hungry or too full. Avoid light, particularly blue light after bedtime. Eliminating a bedside clock or noisy, thrashing bed partner is also recommended. If sleep is not

TABLE 28.1	**Changes in Pregnancy**
Increased Risk of OSA	*Decreased Risk of OSA*
Gestational weight gain	Increased minute ventilation
Nasopharyngeal edema	Lateral sleep position
Decreased functional residual capacity (FRC)	Decreased REM
Hypertension and diabetes	

achieved in 15–20 minutes, leaving the bed to do a simple task that does not increase stress helps change the mindset, facilitating sleep. The only hypnotic medication in pregnancy that is still schedule B is diphenhydramine, although herbal teas and melatonin can also be useful. All other hypnotics are schedule C or lower.

In this patient, the complaint of leg discomfort also needs to be addressed. Leg symptoms are very common in pregnancy, with estimates at 20–40% of pregnant woman experiencing new-onset restless legs in the second half, improving soon after delivery.

Restless leg syndrome requires the occurrence of an urge to move the legs, usually accompanied by a feeling of tingling or discomfort beginning in the evening or night that compels the sufferer to move or walk. It is relieved by movement and may recur with rest.[6] It happens in 5–10% of the general population and may be sporadic or frequent. As it progresses, the arms may be involved. It can happen during periods of prolonged inactivity such as during a plane ride or at a Wagner opera. Disturbed sleep is common, with 85% of patients with RLS reporting periodic movements of sleep as well. When patients who never had RLS become pregnant, 12.5% will have it in the first trimester, and 23% by the third.[7]

There is an important association of RLS with low serum ferritin <18 ng/ml, but levels under 50 ng/ml, while within normal limits, may cause symptoms and should be treated. Ferrous sulfate 325 mg plus vitamin C to enhance absorption, 100 mg one hour before meals, is suggested up to three times per day. It is recommended to measure serum iron, ferritin, and TIBC to rule out hemochromatosis. Nonmedical therapies include massage, stretching, a hot bath, a vibrating bed mat, and venodyne like leg pressure cuff (not tested in pregnancy).

All of the commonly used RLS medications—pramipexole, ropinirole, gabapentin, pregabalin, clonazepam—are schedule C or lower. Oxycodone is the only schedule B medication, and a low dose of 2.5–5 mg may be very effective in refractory patients. In some patients, especially if leg cramps are an issue, 250–400 mg magnesium may be useful.

Recommendations

Sleep hygiene discussion, testing for and treating sleep apnea if found, and measurement of serum ferritin with treatment of restless legs should bring an improvement in her sleep.

KEY POINTS TO REMEMBER

- Take a sleep history to include time to fall asleep, sleep interruption, duration, snoring, and daytime tiredness.
- Ask specifically about restless leg symptoms in the evening in all pregnant patients.
- Encourage a restful sleep ritual with at least eight hours of time without interruption allotted for sleep.

References

1. National Sleep Foundation. Sleep in America poll 1998. In http://wwwsleepfoundation.org accessed June 14, 2016.
2. Pien GW, Schwab RJ. Sleep disorders in pregnancy. *Sleep*. 2004;27(7):1405–1415.
3. Franklin KA, Holmgren PA, Johnson F, et al. Snoring in pregnancy induced hypertension and growth retardation of the fetus. *Chest*. 2000;117:137–141.
4. Reid J, Taylor-Gjevre R, Gjeve J, et al. Can gestational hypertension be modified by treating nocturnal airflow limitation? *J Clin Sleep Med*. 2013;8(4):311–316.
5. American Academy of Sleep Medicine. *International Classification of Sleep Disorders*. 3rd ed. Darien, IL: American Academy of Sleep Medicine; 2014.
6. Allen RP, Walters AS, Montplaisir J, et al. Restless leg syndrome. Prevalence and impact. REST general population study. *Arch Intern Med*. 2005;165(11):1286–1292.
7. Suzuki K, Ohida T, Sone T, et al. The prevalence of restless leg syndrome among pregnant women in Japan. *Sleep*. 2003;26(6):673–677.

29 Convulsion in a Pregnant Woman

Eudocia Q. Lee

A 31-year-old right-handed woman, who is 19 weeks' pregnant with her second child, presents with her first generalized tonic-clonic seizure. She was in her usual state of good health when her husband awoke at night to find her body shaking in a rhythmic manner. By the time emergency medical services arrived, she was no longer shaking but was confused with no recollection of the event. She vomited twice in the ambulance ride to the hospital. She has no past medical history and has had no difficulty to date with her current or past pregnancies. Her medication list includes only prenatal vitamins. On examination in the emergency department, her vital signs are stable. Her neurological examination reveals slowed finger movements on the left but no other focal neurological deficits. A non-contrast head CT showed a right frontal hypodensity with mass effect concerning for a tumor. She was started on Keppra for seizure management.

What do you do now?

BRAIN TUMOR PRESENTING DURING PREGNANCY

This patient's presentation is not unusual for a brain tumor, but what makes her case complex is her pregnancy. Brain tumors are rare during pregnancy, with an estimated incidence of 3.6 cases of malignant brain tumors per million live births. Maternal and perinatal outcomes from brain tumors have not been systematically reviewed. Extrapolating from the systemic cancer literature and from case reports in brain tumor patients, pregnant women with cancer (including brain tumors) should be considered at high risk for perinatal complications and should seek specialized perinatal care. Indeed, a retrospective series of 215 women with invasive cancers diagnosed during pregnancy, many of whom received treatment with surgery, radiation, and/or chemotherapy, found a higher proportion of small-for-gestation-age children and higher rate of preterm deliveries. Of the 180 pregnancies that did not end in miscarriage or abortion, only 45.8% of children were born at term (≥37 weeks).

MRI is the imaging modality of choice for most brain tumors. The risks associated with *noncontrast* MRIs are generally considered acceptable at any stage of pregnancy. However, gadolinium contrast crosses the placenta and is teratogenic at high and repeated doses in animal studies. Although teratogenic effects have not been observed in the small studies of pregnant women, the American College of Radiology recommends avoiding intravenous gadolinium during pregnancy. If the risk–benefit analysis strongly favors imaging, MRI with gadolinium could be considered, preferably in the third trimester. In this case, because the presence of contrast enhancement suggests a more aggressive tumor and might guide surgical management, this patient (in her second trimester of pregnancy) underwent a brain MRI with gadolinium after discussion with the maternal-fetal medicine team. This revealed a nonenhancing, expansile mass in the right frontal lobe (Figure 29.1).

The optimal management of pregnant women with brain tumors is not known. In non-pregnant patients, surgery is recommended to establish pathology. Case series suggest that neurosurgery for various indications, including brain tumors, may be feasible during pregnancy. Risks to the fetus during neurosurgery include compromised blood flow and oxygenation to the fetus from maternal hypotension, uterine artery vasoconstriction, maternal hypoxemia, acid-base changes, as well as direct effects from anesthesia and analgesics. Consultation with an obstetrician and obstetric anesthesiologist is recommended prior to surgery in the event of possible fetal compromise during surgery.

This patient underwent a resection, but a gross total resection could not be achieved due to the proximity of the tumor to the patient's motor strip. Pathology

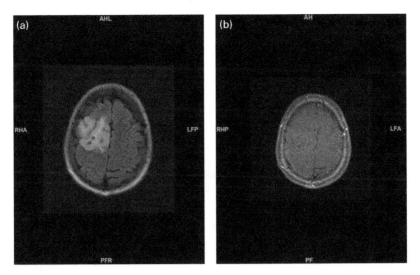

FIGURE 29.1 FLAIR (A) and T1 post-contrast (B) images demonstrate an nonenhancing, expansile mass in the right frontal lobe.

showed a grade 2 oligodendroglioma, considered generally slower growing and less aggressive than higher grade gliomas, but still not curable. Fortunately, molecular testing of her oligodendroglioma demonstrated features associated with longer survival, including an isocitrate dehydrogenase 1 (IDH1) mutation and codeletion of 1p and 19q. With aggressive treatment including surgery, radiation, and chemotherapy, median survival for grade 2 oligodendroglioma ranges from 7–15 years.

Results from a phase 2 trial of patients with low-grade gliomas at higher risk of recurrence (because of older age or because their tumor cannot be completely resected) suggest that such patients should receive adjuvant radiation and chemotherapy. The timing of radiation and chemotherapy after surgery is controversial for patients with relatively good prognoses, such as this patient with an IDH1-mutant, 1p/19q codeleted low-grade oligodendroglioma. In addition, radiation and chemotherapy are generally considered incompatible with fetal health. Depending on the stage of pregnancy, risks to the fetus from radiation include cancer, malformations, mental retardation, and intrauterine death. When chemotherapy is given in the first trimester, the frequency of fetal malformations ranges from 14–19%; the frequency decreases to 1.3% during the second and third trimesters. This patient decided to delay treatment while pregnant.

Her pregnancy and delivery were carefully monitored by a multidisciplinary team including obstetrics, maternal-fetal medicine, anesthesiology, and neurology. Even in normal pregnancy, there are prominent increases in intracranial pressure during labor and vaginal delivery with uterine contractions, pain, and bearing down. As she was clinically stable and her brain tumor had mostly been debulked, she delivered a healthy baby boy without complications.

More than one year now from her presentation, this patient continues to do well and has elected to remain on observation with serial imaging. She understands that her tumor will grow in the future and will ultimately require further treatment. Although she had previously wanted a large family, she is not sure if she will have more children, given the limited prognosis associated with this diagnosis. There are conflicting data as to whether pregnancy accelerates glioma growth. Gliomas, including oligodendrogliomas, are more common in men than in women, with an incidence rate of 1.3:1. Of the primary brain tumors, only meningiomas and pituitary tumors are more common in women than in men.

In summary, brain tumors are rare during pregnancy but can be complex to manage and require multidisciplinary care. Chemotherapy and radiation are associated with congenital malformations and other untoward effects on the fetus, and therefore treatment plans often need to take into account both the mother and the fetus. Fertility preservation is also an important issue in young women with brain tumors who may require chemotherapy and/or radiation.

KEY POINTS TO REMEMBER

- Of the primary brain tumors, meningiomas and pituitary tumors are more common in women than in men.
- The care of pregnant women with primary brain tumors requires a multidisciplinary approach involving obstetrics, maternal-fetal medicine, neurosurgery, anesthesiology, neurology, medical oncology, and radiation oncology.
- Chemotherapy and radiation are generally considered incompatible with normal fetal development.
- The risks associated with noncontrast MRIs are generally considered acceptable at any stage of pregnancy, although intravenous gadolinium should be avoided if possible during pregnancy.

References

Haas JF, Janisch W, Staneczek W. Newly diagnosed primary intracranial neoplasms in pregnant women: a population-based assessment. *J Neurol Neurosurg Psychiatry*. 1986;49:874–880.

Van Calsteren K, Heyns L, De Smet F, et al. Cancer during pregnancy: an analysis of 215 patients emphasizing the obstetrical and the neonatal outcomes. *J Clin Oncol.* 2010;28:683–689.

Schiff D. Low-grade gliomas. *Continuum (Minneap Minn).* 2015;21:345–354.

Buckner JC, Shaw EG, Pugh SL, et al. Radiation plus procarbazine, CCNU, and vincristine in low-grade glioma. *N Engl J Med.* 2016;374:1344–1355.

Yust-Katz S, de Groot JF, Liu D, et al. Pregnancy and glial brain tumors. *Neuro-Oncology.* 2014;16:1289–1294.

Women's Health and Aging

30 Cognitive Concerns

M. Angela O'Neal

A 50-year-old woman whose mother has Alzheimer's disease (AD) is concerned about getting the disorder. She is healthy, without any significant medical problems. Her only medications are calcium and vitamin D. Her neurological examination is normal. She asks about whether she should be on hormone replacement therapy.

What do you do now?

ALZHEIMER'S DISEASE

Incidence

The incidence of AD increases with age. In fact, the frequency of dementia doubles every five years beginning at age 60. The prevalence has increased such that one in nine people over age 65 have AD. AD disproportionately affects women. Women make up two-thirds of the caregivers for the disorder. In addition, AD is two to three times more common in women, which is not explained by women's longer life expectancy.

Role of Hormonal Replacement

Observational trials suggested that estrogen could play a role in delaying the onset of AD. However, the Women's Health Initiative Memory Study (WHIMS), published in 2003, demonstrated that estrogen, with or without medroxyprogesterone, substantially increased their risk of dementia of any cause, with AD being the most frequent etiology. This was a randomized controlled trial with two study arms, one involving 4532 postmenopausal women over age 65 who received continuous combined estrogen plus medroxyprogesterone acetate or placebo, and the other involving 2947 hysterectomized women randomized to continuous unopposed combined estrogen or placebo. Overall, the risk of probable dementia for women in the estrogen plus progestin group was twice that of women in the placebo group, and the increased risk began to appear as early as one year after randomization.[1]

That the timing of hormone replacement might be important was raised with an observational trial of 1768 women followed from 1995 to 2006 in Cache County, Utah. Detailed information was obtained regarding age of menopause and hormonal therapy (HT). The population-based study showed that women who used HT within five years of menopause had a 30% lower risk of AD, especially if the use of HT lasted longer than 10 years.[2] These observational results were not supported with a recent trial. The trial randomized women within six years or more than 10 years of menopause to receive estrogen hormonal therapy or placebo. The results showed that estrogen did not benefit or harm cognitive function regardless of the time post menopause.[3]

Gender Risk

There have been some interesting findings that may explain why women may be more susceptible to AD. It is known that the apolipoprotein E genotype with the (APOE∈4) allele represents a major risk factor for AD. Farrer et al. found that the risk of AD associated with a given genotype varies with sex. Women who had either the ∈4/∈4 or ∈3/∈4 genotype were at higher risk to develop AD than men with the same genotype.[4] Data from the Harvard Aging Brain Study show that women are more likely than men to accumulate amyloid and so have a larger amyloid burden when adjusted by age. This sex difference in AD is also seen in response to medication. Women with similar age, functional status, cognitive scores, and duration of AD show a more rapid cognitive decline than men treated with donepezil.

Prevention

There is no current prevention for AD. The recommendation to the patient is that there is no role for HT in AD prevention. She should maintain a regular exercise program, a heart-healthy diet, and continue with brain-stimulating activities such as new learning and active socialization.

KEY POINTS TO REMEMBER

1. Alzheimer's disease is two to three times more common in women than in men.
2. There is no role for hormone therapy in AD prevention or treatment.
3. Current best prevention of AD includes a healthy diet, active exercise program, and brain-stimulation activities.

References

1. Shumaker SA, Legault C, Rapp S, et al. Estrogen plus progestin and the incidence of dementia and mild cognitive impairment in postmenopausal women: The Women's Health Initiative Memory Study: a randomized controlled trial. *JAMA*. 2003;289:2651–2662.
2. Shao H, Breitner JCS, Whitmer RA, et al. Hormone therapy and Alzheimer disease dementia: new findings from the Cache County Study. *Neurology*. 2012;79(18):1846–1852.
3. Henderson VW, St John JA, Hodis HN, et al. Cognitive effects of estradiol after menopause: A randomized trial of the timing hypothesis. *Neurology*. 2016 Aug 16;87(7):699–708.
4. Farrer LA, Cupples LA, Haines JL, et al. Effects of age, sex, and ethnicity on the association between apolipoprotein E genotype and Alzheimer disease: a meta-analysis. *JAMA*. 1997;278(16):1349–1356.

31 "Will I Have a Stroke?"

M. Angela O'Neal

A 76-year-old woman with a history of diabetes mellitus
(DM), hypertension, and new-onset atrial fibrillation (AF)
is referred for evaluation of her stroke risk. She does
not smoke and drinks one or two alcoholic beverages a
week. She has never had a TIA or stroke. She had a twin
pregnancy at age 28 complicated by eclampsia. Her exam
is normal.

What do you do now?

STROKE

Incidence

Stroke in women is the third leading cause of death. One in five women will have a stroke. Age-adjusted stroke risks can be misleading as they do not speak to the burden of stroke. Men do have a higher incidence of stroke across most age ranges. However, in the population over 85, women have a higher or similar risk of stroke, and as women live longer than men, their stroke burden is substantial.

Gender-Specific Risk Factors

Preeclampsia/Eclampsia

A growing body of literature supports the fact that complications of pregnancy are associated with higher risk of future cerebrovascular disease beyond pregnancy. For example, women with a history of preeclampsia have 2–10-fold risk of developing chronic hypertension, which is a powerful risk factor for stroke. Fifty percent of women with gestational DM will develop type II DM within five to 10 years of their pregnancy. (1,2) Pregnancy acts as a "stress test," in that women who are likely to develop vascular dysfunction often do so initially during pregnancy. Multiple retrospective cohort studies have demonstrated that preeclampsia and eclampsia increase stroke risk. The consensus is that women who have preeclampsia have twice the risk of stroke and a four-fold risk of high blood pressure later in life.

Atrial Fibrillation

Two large cohort studies have confirmed an age–gender interaction in women with AF. In women with AF over the age of 75, there is a higher risk of stroke than in men. For example, in a large study of over 100,000 patients with non-valvular AF in Sweden, the incident risk of stroke was greater in women than in men (6.2% vs. 4.2% per year). (3) Recent scales to estimate stroke risk related to AF take these gender and age differences into account.

Guidelines

The differences in stroke risk in women prompted the American Heart and Stroke Association in 2014 to publish a guideline to stroke prevention in women. (4) They defined stroke risk factors that are sex-specific, such as pregnancy, pre-eclampsia, gestational diabetes, oral contraceptive use, and postmenopausal hormone use. In addition, there are several conditions associated with stroke that are more common in women, including migraine with aura, AF, DM, and hypertension. The authors concluded that, to accurately reflect the risk of stroke in women, a female-specific stroke risk score is warranted.

Recommendations for Our Patient

Our patient should have her DM and hypertension aggressively treated. A baseline fasting lipid profile was ordered. Her goal low-density lipoprotein level, taking into account her multiple risk factors, should be less than 100 mg/dl. As regards the atrial fibrillation, she has a high risk of having embolic events. The factors that increase the embolic risk include her age, gender, DM, and hypertension. Therefore, initiating anticoagulation was recommended. She has nonvalvular AF, so either warfarin or a factor Xa inhibitor could be used.

KEY POINTS TO REMEMBER

1. Stroke is the third leading cause of death in women.
2. Stroke risk factors that are unique to women include: preeclampsia/eclampsia, gestational DM, and oral contraceptive use.
3. Migraine with aura, AF, DM, and hypertension are stroke risk factors that are more common in women.

References

1. Funai EF, Friedlander Y, Paltiel O, et al. Long-term mortality after preeclampsia. *Epidemiology*. 2005;16:206–215.
2. Mannisto T, Mendola P, Vaarasmaki M, et al. Elevated blood pressure in pregnancy and subsequent chronic disease risk. *Circulation*. 2013;127:681–690.
3. Friberg L, Rosenqvist M, Lip GHY. Evaluation of risk stratification schemes for ischaemic stroke and bleeding in 182 678 patients with atrial fibrillation: the Swedish Atrial Fibrillation cohort study. *European Heart Journal*. 2012;33:1500–1510.
4. Bushnell C, McCullough LD, Awad IA, et al. Guidelines for the Prevention of Stroke in Women: a statement for healthcare professionals from the American Heart Association/American Stroke Association. *Stroke*. 2014;45:1–35.

32 Involuntary Movements

Chizoba Umeh

A 69-year-old woman presents to the neurology clinic for evaluation of involuntary movements. She has a 19-year history of Parkinson's disease (PD) and history of hypertension, hyperlipidemia, and peripheral arterial disease. She developed involuntary choreiform movements of the head, trunk, and limbs, gradually worsening over the past five years. The involuntary movements occur during 50% of her waking hours and result in fatigue. Her medications for PD include carbidopa/levodopa/entacapone, rasagiline, ropinirole, and amantadine.

On exam, she has a blood pressure of 130/58 and pulse of 77. She has decreased facial expression, reduced voice volume, and cogwheel rigidity in the upper extremities. Her gait is stooped and severely slowed with freezing steps. She has severe-intensity choreiform movements of the face, trunk, and legs.

What do you do now?

LEVODOPA-INDUCED DYSKINESIA

The term *chorea*, stemming from the Greek word for dance ("choreia") describes brief, irregular, non-rhythmic, flowing, involuntary movements. In a patient presenting with choreic movements, the differential diagnosis is broad and includes hereditary causes of chorea such as Huntington's disease and Wilson's disease, in addition to acquired causes (stroke, paraneoplastic, infectious, drug-induced). There is no family history in this case to support a hereditary etiology. The slow clinical course argues against an acute vascular etiology such as an infarct or hemorrhage. If focal neurological signs are present, MRI of the brain should be considered to rule out a lesion in the basal ganglia. Vascular causes of chorea can often result in contralateral hemichorea or hemiballismus as opposed to generalized chorea.

A brain MRI in this patient showed incidental finding of moderate white matter disease of the cerebral hemispheres and pons consistent with chronic microvascular ischemic disease.

If there is family history of chorea, genetic testing can be considered as part of the workup. In younger patients presenting with chorea, tremor, and psychiatric symptoms, serum copper/ceruloplasmin, liver function tests, and 24-hour urine copper may be obtained as initial evaluation for Wilson's disease.

The patient's history of neurodegenerative PD and chronic levodopa treatment is an important clue that the likely cause of the movement disorder is levodopa-induced involuntary choreic movements, also termed "dyskinesia." Patients often report "peak dose dyskinesia" in the evening when the total daily levodopa dose accumulates and the dyskinesia may be the most severe.

It is important to note that not all Parkinson's patients on levodopa therapy develop dyskinesia. Certain risk factors have been identified: younger age of onset of PD, greater disease severity, higher levodopa dose, and longer duration of levodopa treatment. For unclear reasons, women have been shown in some studies to be more likely to develop dyskinesia.

Patients can have varying severity of dyskinesia. The decision to treat the dyskinesia depends on the degree of disability to the patient. While some patients exhibit anosognosia, and are unaware of the dyskinesia, others have severe, disabling dyskinesia that may impact their coordination, gait, and quality of life.

For patients with troublesome dyskinesia, various treatments options are available. One approach is to decrease the likelihood of peak dose dyskinesia by lowering the per-dose amount of levodopa (i.e., reduce from 200 mg to 150 mg per dose) while increasing the number of times the levodopa therapy is taken daily (i.e., from three times daily to four times daily). Amantadine, an antiviral and antiparkinsonian agent, has shown efficacy in reducing dyskinesia. Intraduodenal levodopa directly delivers levodopa to the duodenum and jejunum and has been shown to reduce dyskinesia. Surgical treatment with placement of a deep brain stimulator in the subthalamic nucleus or globus pallidus interna is another approach to managing dyskinesia. This patient received a deep brain stimulator to the globus pallidus interna with reduction of the dyskinesia.

Once levodopa-induced dyskinesia develops, it generally remains present at varying frequency and severity, depending on the daily dose of levodopa and adjunctive treatments for PD.

KEY POINTS TO REMEMBER

- Choreiform involuntary movements, "dyskinesia," are a manifestation of chronic levodopa treatment in PD.
- Vascular causes such as infarct or hemorrhage should be excluded in patients with acute onset hemi-chorea.
- Pharmacological or surgical treatment should be considered in PD patients with disabling dyskinesia.

References

1. Warren Olanow C, Kieburtz K, Rascol O, et al. Factors predictive of the development of levodopa-induced dyskinesia and wearing-off in Parkinson's disease. *Mov Disord*. 2013;28:1064–1071.

2. Thanvi B, Lo N, Robinson T. Levodopa-induced dyskinesia in Parkinson's disease: clinical features, pathogenesis, prevention and treatment. *Postgrad Med J*. 2007;83:384–388.

3. Mazzucchi S, Frosini D, Bonuccelli U, Ceravolo R. Current treatment and future prospects of dopa-induced dyskinesias. *Drugs Today (Barcelona)*. 2015;51:315–329.

4. Lundqvist C. Continuous levodopa for advanced Parkinson's disease. *Neuropsychiatric Dis Treat*. 2007;3:335–3348.

33 Memory Concerns in Middle Age

Marie Pasinski

A 48 year old teacher confides, "I can't remember words or names. Eventually it comes to me, but I'm worried I'm developing Alzheimer's, like my mother." She has not made any errors at work, oversees the care of her mother, and continues to manage her own family's household and finances without difficulty. She denies any other neurological symptoms. Her recent history is notable for a 10 lb. weight gain over the past year in the setting of perimenopause, poor sleep, and dysthymia.

Her past medical history is remarkable for borderline hypertension and glucose intolerance. She takes over-the-counter (OTC) diphenhydramine to help her sleep but otherwise is not on any medications. She drinks two to three glasses of wine per night. She does not smoke cigarettes or marijuana, or use illicit drugs. She does not exercise.

Physical exam is notable for BP 148/90 and BMI of 32.5. Her neurological exam is normal, including mental status and the Montreal Cognitive Assessment (MOCA).

What do you do now?

IMPROVING COGNITION THROUGH LIFESTYLE CHANGES

Memory concerns and word-finding difficulties in middle age are extremely common, typically benign, and can be improved by lifestyle modification. Although this patient performed well on cognitive testing, she has multiple dementia risk factors, which, if addressed, could improve her cognitive functioning both in the short term and in the long run.

While we cannot change our genes, new research suggests that lifestyle changes can decrease our risk of Alzheimer's, the most common cause of dementia, through epigenetic alteration of gene function. One-third of Alzheimer's cases are estimated to be attributable to seven modifiable risk factors, including: diabetes, hypertension, obesity, smoking, depression, cognitive inactivity, and physical inactivity.[1] In addition, sleep disorders are now a recognized risk factor for dementia. Perhaps more importantly, studies show that lifestyle interventions can improve cognitive performance. A promising randomized controlled trial, the Finnish Geriatric Intervention Study to Prevent Cognitive Impairment and Disability (FINGER), showed that a multidomain intervention of diet, exercise, cognitive training, and vascular risk monitoring significantly improved cognitive performance, including tests of executive function and memory.[2]

Seven Steps to Optimize Brain Health

Assess General Health

Virtually every organ system supports brain function. Neurologists witness this regularly when consulting on patients with mental status change. The most common cause is metabolic encephalopathy. Even minor deviations in brain homeostasis can have profound effects on cognition both in the short term and in the long run. For example, pulmonary, cardiac, respiratory, hepatic, renal, immune, and endocrine disturbances can all secondarily impair cognitive function. Maintaining good blood flow to the brain is especially key. Consequently, special attention should be given to diabetes, hypertension, and other vascular risk factors that compromise brain blood flow. Maximizing general health and aggressively treating underlying medical conditions is crucial to achieving optimal brain health. A common screen for cognitive concerns may include the following: Complete blood count (CBC), , a comprehensive metabolic profile (CMP), thyroid screening panel, vitamin B_{12}, folate, syphilis, human immunodeficiency virus (HIV), and neuroimaging.

Review Medications (Including OTCs), Alcohol and Tobacco History

Be aware that medications, particularly those that are psychoactive and cross the blood–brain barrier can impair memory and cognition. Chronic use of benzodiazepines and anticholinergics such as diphenhydramine (commonly used as sleeping aids as in the previous example) have been associated with an increased risk of dementia. Keep in mind that alcohol is toxic to neurons, and the current thinking is that drinking less is better when it comes to brain health. For women, intake should be limited to no more than one standard alcoholic drink per day. Smoking is a significant risk factor for Alzheimer's and should be discouraged.

Address Weight and Diet

Midlife obesity is an established risk factor for Alzheimer's disease. Comorbidities including hypertension, decreased physical activity from osteoarthritis, and diabetes, may be contributing factors. In addition, even in those who are not diabetic, insulin resistance may be important and negatively affect brain energy metabolism, amyloid clearance, and memory formation.

Numerous large observational studies support the "Mediterranean diet" as the best diet to decrease the risk of dementia and improve cognition. The new kid on the block is the MIND diet (Mediterranean-DASH Intervention for Neurodegenerative Delay) which is a combination of the Mediterranean diet and the Dietary Approaches to Stop Hypertension (DASH) diet. The DASH diet, which is naturally low in sodium and high in potassium, has been shown to lower blood pressure. The DASH diet is rich in fruits, vegetables, whole grains, and low-fat dairy foods; includes meat, fish, poultry, nuts, and beans; and is limited in sugar-sweetened foods and beverages, red meat, and added fat. The MIND diet provides parameters of 10 healthy foods to be eaten regularly and five unhealthy foods to be avoided (see Table 33.1). Study participants who followed this diet for an average of four years had a 54% decreased risk of Alzheimer's disease when the diet was followed rigorously, and a 35% decreased risk of Alzheimer's when followed moderately.[3]

Take a Sleep History

Sleep deprivation and sleep disorders are a recognized risk factor for Alzheimer's disease. Sleep-disordered breathing is associated with twice the odds of developing dementia. Additionally, irregular circadian rhythms increase the risk of dementia and mild cognitive impairment (MCI). This may be related to our new understanding that neurogenesis and neuroplastic changes occur during sleep. Fascinating functional MRI (fMRI) studies demonstrate that new information and skills learned during the day are reorganized during sleep. More recently, studies show that beta-amyloid, which forms the pathological amyloid plaques in Alzheimer's disease, is cleared from the brain during sleep.

TABLE 33.1 **MIND Diet Guidelines**

10 Brain Healthy Foods	5 Unhealthy Foods to Avoid
Green leafy vegetables: 6 servings/week	***Red meat:*** Less than 4 servings/week
Other vegetables: 1 or more servings/day	***Butter and margarine:*** Less than 1 Tbsp./day
Nuts: 5 servings/week	***Cheese:*** Less than 1 serving/week
Berries: 2 or more servings/week	***Pastries and sweets:*** Less than 5 servings/week
Beans: 3 or more servings/week	***Fried or fast food:*** Less than 1 serving/week
Whole grains: 3 or more servings/day	
Fish: 1 serving/week	
Poultry: 2 servings/week	
Olive oil: Use as your main cooking oil	
Wine: 1 glass a day	

When proper sleep hygiene does not correct insomnia or fragmented sleep, consider a sleep study or referral to a sleep specialist.

Encourage Physical Activity

Exercise is one of the most potent ways to improve brain health, while physical inactivity is considered to be the number one modifiable risk factor for Alzheimer's disease in the United States. Physical activity causes the release of brain-derived neurotrophic factor (BDNF), nicknamed "Miracle-Gro for the Brain," which promotes synaptic plasticity and neurogenesis. Low levels of BDNF have been associated with cognitive decline.

Numerous studies have shown that regular aerobic exercise increases brain volume on MRI volumetric brain imaging. Most notably, the size of the hippocampus, the center of memory and learning, becomes more robust when sedentary individuals engage in progressive aerobic training. There also is a very strong correlation between physical fitness and improved cognitive functioning.

Screen for Depression and Anxiety

Depressed adults over age 50 are 65% more likely to develop Alzheimer's compared to those without depression. Although this association does not establish a cause, depression and anxiety are interestingly associated with increased levels of stress hormones and lower levels of BDNF—both of which have been shown to inhibit hippocampal neurogenesis. Screening for these conditions and instituting proper treatment can improve quality of life and may, in turn, improve cognitive functioning.

Promote Mental Challenge

Higher educational attainment and engagement in mentally challenging activities throughout life are associated with improved cognitive function and lower rates of dementia. The brain has the ability to make new neurons and new synapses throughout our lives. This process is stimulated by mental challenge and, like exercise, releases brain growth factors, including BDNF.

During our youth when we are constantly exposed to new concepts, new experiences, and new learning, this system is in overdrive. As we get older and set in our routines, mental stimulation often wanes. However, there is no physiological reason that we cannot continue to challenge our intellect with new experiences and new learning throughout our lives and reap the benefits of lifelong learning.

KEY POINTS TO REMEMBER

- Alzheimer's disease can be prevented or delayed.
- One-third of cases of Alzheimer's disease are attributed to modifiable lifestyle risk factors.
- Lifestyle interventions have been shown to improve cognitive performance and decrease the risk of Alzheimer's.

References

1. Norton S, Matthews FE, Barnes DE, et al. Potential for primary prevention of Alzheimer's disease: an analysis of populationbased data base. *Lancet Neurol.* 2014;13:788–794.

2. Ngandu T. A 2-year multidomain intervention of diet, exercise, cognitive training, and vascular risk monitoring versus control to prevent cognitive decline in at risk elderly people (FINGER): a randomized controlled trial. *Lancet.* 2015;385(9984):2255–2263.

3. Morris MC, Tangney CC, Wang Y, et al. MIND diet associated with reduced incidence of Alzheimer's disease. *Alzheimers Dement.* 2015 Sep;11(9):1007–1014.

34 Pain in the Back

M. Angela O'Neal

A 56-year-old woman is referred for evaluation of focal with secondary generalized epilepsy. She has a long history of epilepsy since her teens. Her seizure are typically episodes of staring with some lip smacking, following which she is confused and sleepy for 10 minutes. Occasionally the seizures are generalized with tonic-clonic movements and a more prolonged confusional period of 20–30 minutes. She has been on a stable dose of phenytoin for many years. Her brain MRI is normal, and a past electroencephalogram (EEG) showed occasional right temporal sharp waves. Her last seizure was over a year ago, in the setting of missing several doses of phenytoin.

While carrying a heavy box, she developed severe low back pain. Her internist did a lumbar spine film, which showed an L1 compression fracture.

Her only medication is phenytoin 300 mg at night.

Her back exam is normal. On neurological exam, there is changing direction nystagmus on both directions of lateral gaze.

What do you do now?

EFFECTS OF NEUROLOGICAL DRUGS ON BONE HEALTH

Osteoporosis is a skeletal disorder where decreased bone strength leads to fractures. Antiepileptic drugs, AEDs, are known to affect bone metabolism. This is especially true for those that induce the cytochrome P450 system. Activation of the P450 system causes increased breakdown of vitamin D. This in turn leads to less gastrointestinal absorption of calcium, which stimulates elevated levels of parathyroid hormone. Parathyroid hormone increases lead to more calcium mobilization from bone and increased bone turnover.[1]

Specific AEDs and Bone Health

The enzyme-inducing AEDs include phenytoin, carbamazepine, phenobarbital, and primidone. Valproate is not an enzyme inducer. However, it is reported to increase both the rate of bone loss and fracture incidence. This appears to be correlated with dose and duration of valproate therapy. Clonazepam and Oxcarbazepine also have an associated small increased risk of fractures. There is no data on the carbonic anhydrase inhibitors, topiramate and zonisamide. Studies on lamotrigine and levetiracetam have demonstrated no adverse effects on bone mineral density.[2,3]

Risk Factors for Osteoporosis

Risk factors for osteoporosis have been well studied. They include: female gender, postmenopausal state, inactivity, low body mass, chronic illness, inadequate vitamin D and calcium intake, limited sunlight exposure, and smoking. Additional risk factors for osteoporosis in patients with epilepsy include the type and number of AEDs and the duration of therapy.

Epilepsy and Fall Risk

Patients with epilepsy have a higher fall risk, both directly due to the epilepsy as well as to the AED effect on gait stability. This is especially true for individuals who have generalized epilepsy and those on multiple-drug regimens. In the Woman's Health Initiative study, which followed women ages 50–79 on AEDs and those not on an AED, the use of AEDs was clearly associated with a significant increase in risk of fractures. Fracture risk is related to the epilepsy type, the degree of control of the epilepsy, and the drug regimen, including which AEDs are used, their dose, and the duration of therapy.[4]

Screening

Osteoporosis screening with a bone mineral density scan (BMD) is recommended for postmenopausal women and those with additional risk factors. In women with epilepsy, the risks of AED use as well as the risks related to fall put them at even higher risk. It is reasonable to screen with a BMD in women with epilepsy who have additional risk factors for osteoporosis. In epileptics on an AED, it is recommended to check serum calcium, phosphate, and 25-hydroxy vitamin D levels.[5]

Prevention

The usual lifestyle recommendations should be also be made: regular weight-bearing exercise and smoking cessation. Low calcium or vitamin D levels should be replaced. Adequate calcium doses in older adults, 1200 mg daily, and vitamin D 400–800 U daily, are recommended. Consideration about changing the AED regimen needs to be individualized and weighed against the risk of recurrent seizure.

KEY POINTS TO REMEMBER

1. AEDs, particularly those that are enzyme-inducing, increase the risk of osteoporosis.
2. Patients with epilepsy have a higher fall risk.
3. Patients at risk for osteoporosis should be screened with a BMD.
4. Calcium and vitamin D supplementation are important in patients with epilepsy to support bone health.

References

1. Pack AM. Bone disease in epilepsy. *Curr Neurol Neurosci Rep*. 2004;4:329–334.
2. Pack AM, Morrell MJ, Marcus R, et al. Bone mass and turnover in women with epilepsy on antiepileptic drug monotherapy. *Ann Neurol*. 2005;57:252–257.
3. Mintzer S, Boppana P, Toguri J, DeSantis A. Vitamin D levels and bone turnover in epilepsy patients taking carbamazepine or oxcarbazepine. *Epilepsia*. 2006;47:510–515.
4. Vestergaard P, Tigaran S, Rejnmark L, et al. Fracture risk is increased in epilepsy. *Acta Neurol Scand*. 1999;99:269–275.
5. Meier C, Kraenzlin ME. Antiepileptics and Bone Health. *Ther Adv Musculoskelet Dis*. 2011 Oct;3(5):235–243.

Index

Note: Page numbers followed by b, *f,* or *t* indicate a box, figure, or table respectively

assisted reproductive technology, in MS, 130–131

assisted reproductive technology (ART), in MS, 130–131

atenolol
  migraines and, 6t
  myasthenia gravis and, 123b
  for postpartum migraines, 69t

atrial fibrillation (ATF), 155–157

autoimmune myasthenia gravis, 121

Avonex*, 127

azathioprine, 121, 123t, 137

azithromycin, 123b

B-cell lymphocytopenia, 121

benzodiazepines
  dementia and, 164–165
  for seizure clusters, 26

Bestaseron*, 127

beta blockers
  migraines and, 6t
  myasthenia gravis and, 123b
  for postpartum migraines, 69t

bilateral papilledema, 34

botulinum toxins, 123b

brain-derived neurotropic factor (BDNF), 166, 167

brain health optimization, 164–167
  alcohol, medication, tobacco history, 164–165
  anxiety/depression screening, 166–167
  general health assessment, 164
  mental challenges, 167
  MIND diet guidelines, 166t
  physical activity, 166
  sleep history, 165–166
  weight and diet, 165, 166t

brain MRI, 9, 20. *See also* magnetic resonance imaging
  acute infarct, lenticulostriate territory, 80f
  brain tumor, 144
  CVT, 92
  epilepsy, 29, 169
  idiopathic intracranial hypertension, 72, 72f
  left cerebral artery occlusion, 81f
  migraine, stroke, 21, 21f
  monthly seizures, 25

optic neuritis, 133

Parkinson's disease, 160

posterior reversible encephalopathy syndrome, 85f
  during pregnancy, 64
  thalamic glioblastoma, 35f

brainstem syndromes, 135

brain tumor in pregnancy, 144–146

breast feeding
  AED choice and, 41
  multiple sclerosis and, 125–127, 130–131
  NMOSD and, 138

bromocriptine, 97

buffalo hump, 52

bupivacaine, 103, 106

butalbital, 69t

cabergoline, 47

caesarian section (C-section), 91, 92, 94, 100, 133

calcium, bone health and, 170, 170

calcium channel blockers
  migraines and, 6t
  myasthenia gravis and, 123b
  for RCVS, 89

cancer treatment, infertility and, 35–37

carbamazepine, 170

carbidopa/levodopa/entacapone, 159

carbonic anhydrase inhibitors, 170

carotid endarterectomy, 89

carpal tunnel syndrome, 109–112
  associated conditions, 112
  incidence/causes, 110
  pinprick sensation, 109, 111, 113
  sensory loss in, 111, 111f
  signs and symptoms, 110, 111b
  testing for, 111–112

catamenial epilepsy, 25–27

cauda equina injury, 116b

cerebral lesions, symptomatic, 135

cerebral venous thrombosis (CVT)
  clinical features, 92
  clotting factors in pregnancy, 93f
  future pregnancies and, 93–94
  IIH and, 72
  pathophysiology, 92–93
  treatment, 93, 94

cervical artery dissection, 23
CHC. *See* combined hormonal contraception
chemotherapy
    brain tumors and, 144–146
    for glioblastoma, 35, 36
chloroprocaine, 106
cholinesterase inhibitors, 121
choreiform movements, 159, 161
Chronic Insomnia Disorder (ICD-10-CM
        code: F51.01), 140
clobazem, 26, 27
clonazepam, 170, 141
clopidogrel (Plavix), 105*t*
cocaine, 89
codeine, 69*t*
Colles fracture, 112
combined hormonal contraception (CHC)
    AEDs, interactions with, 12
    ischemic stroke risk with, 4–5
computed tomography (CT)
    frontal head bleed, 100*f*
    myasthenia gravis, 120
    during pregnancy, 65–66
    reversible cerebral vasospasm
        syndrome, 88*f*
    stroke, 66
convulsions, in pregnancy, 143–145
cortical spreading depression (CSD), 22
corticotrophin-releasing hormone (CRH), 52
Cushing's disease, 52–54
    Cushing's syndrome comparison, 52, 54
    description, 52
    diagnosis, 52–53
    female *vs.* male prevalence, 52
Cushing's syndrome
    ACTH-dependent *vs.* -independent, 53
    causes, 54
    comorbidities, 52
    Cushing's disease comparison, 52, 54
    PCOS and, 31
    symptoms, 52
cyclosporine, 121, 122*t*
cytochrome P450 system, 170

DASH (Dietary Approaches to Stop
    Hypertension) diet, 165
deep-brain glioblastoma, 35–36

dementia. *See also* Alzheimer's disease
    exacerbating factors, 164–165
    hormonal replacement risks, 152
    prevalence, 152
    prevention strategies, 33, 164–165
Depakote ER 750, 30
depression screening, 166–167
diabetes insipidus (DI), 97
diabetes mellitus, 155
    gestational, 73, 112, 116, 156, 157
    stroke and, 156–157
    type II, 51, 52, 156
dihydroergotamine, 69*t*
Dijon Stroke Registry, 22
Dilantin, 121
dimethyl fumarate (Tecfidera'), 128*t*
diphenhydramine, 163
disease-modifying therapy (DMT), in MS,
    123, 127–130. *See also* specific agents
diuretics, 73
dopamine agonists, 47, 48
double vision
    epidural anesthesia and, 106
    IIH and, 72
    procatinoma and, 48
dural puncture headache, 106–107. *See also*
    postdural puncture headache
dyskinesia. *See* levodopa-induced dyskinesia

eclampsia
    definition, 84
    ischemic stroke and, 80
    migraines and, 68, 70
    myasthenia gravis and, 121
    pathophysiology, 84
    stroke and, 156
    treatment, 84–85, 88
Ecstasy (XTC), 88
electroencephalogram (EEG), 9, 11*f*
endocrine dysfunction, 97
endocrinopathies, 31
endothelial dysfunction, 84, 85, 88
enoxaparin (Lovenox), 105*t*
enzyme-inducing antiepileptic drugs
    (AEDs), 170. *See also* carbamazepine;
    phenobarbital; phenytoin; primidone
epidural abscess, 105–106

stroke (*Cont.*)
   ischemic, 4–5, 79–82
   migraine-induced, 19–23
   migraine with aura and, 4–5, 17, 23, 156
   transient ischemic, 155
subdural hematoma, 76
succinylcholine, 123b
sumatriptan, 19, 68

tacrolimus, 89
telithromycin, 123b
teratogenic medication, 12, 39–40. *See also*
   topiramate
teratogens, 12. *See also* topiramate
teriflunomide, 128*t*
teriflunomide (Aubagio'), 128*t*, 129
tetralogy of Fallot, 129
thalamic glioblastoma (GMB), 35–36
theophylline, 77
thunderclap headache, 87–89
thymoma, 120
tibial malformation, 129
timolol, 69*t*
timolol maleate eye drops, 123b
tinnitus, 72, 75, 76, 106, 107
tirofiban (Aggrastat), 105*t*
tobacco use history, 164–165
tobramycin, 123b
tonic-clonic seizures, 169, 39, 91, 99, 143
tonsillar herniation syndrome, 76
topiramate (TPM)
   bone health and, 170
   for IGE, 57
   for IIH, 73
   for JME, 11
   migraines and, 5, 6*t*
   pregnancy classification, 13*t*
   for primary epilepsy, 12b, 13b
   side effects, 12
transient ischemic stroke (TIA), 155
transverse myelitis, 135

tricyclic antidepressants, 6*t*
triptans
   for menstrually-related migraines, 17
   for postpartum migraine
      management, 69*t*
   RCVS and, 89
d-tubocurarine, 123b
type II diabetes mellitus, 51, 52, 156
Tysabri Pregnancy Exposure Registry, 129

U.S. Food and Drug Administration
   (FDA), 41, 127
U.S. Health and Human Services, 4

valproate
   bone health and, 170
   for JME, 11–12
   migraines and, 6*t*
   PCOS and, 31–32
   pregnancy classification, 13*t*
valproic acid (VPA), 39–40, 55
vasoactive medications, 89
vecuronium, 123b
verapamil, 6*t*
vitamin B$_{12}$ supplement, 39
vitamin C, 141
vitamin D, 170, 171

Wilson's disease, 160
Women's Health Initiative, 170
Women's Health Initiative Memory Study
   (WHIMS), 152
Women's Health Study (WHS), 5
women with epilepsy (WWE), 56
World Health Organization (WHO), 22

zolmitriptan, 17
zonisamide
   bone health and, 170
   for generalized epilepsy, 12
   pregnancy classification, 13*t*